# Healing Devotions

Steps toward being healed
and walking in **Divine Health**

by Patricia L. Whipp

By Patricia L. Whipp

# Healing Devotions

ISBN 10:   1-947714-00-7
ISBN 13:   978-1-947714-00-7

**The Printed Word**
PO Box 7734
La Verne, CA 91750

*Words of*

*Teaching*

*Encouragement*

*and*

*Strength to Stand*

*for Healing*

By Patricia L. Whipp

# January 1

**God wants you healed.** Your healing has been bought and paid for. Jesus went to the cross for your healing. By His stripes you are healed. The Amplified Bible even says you were made whole.

God ordained this for you. He saw His Son suffer. So when He sees you sick, He sees your healing bought and paid for. What a horrible price.

Do not ever think that God wants you sick. He will take advantage of having your attention and will teach you things, but He would rather teach you when you are well!

Study your Bible. Learn scriptures that tell you that God has provided healing for you.

Learn to thank God for your health. He has provided it for you. It is always good to praise and thank God.

> Isaiah 53:5 - But He was wounded for our transgressions, He was bruised for our iniquities; the chastisement for our peace was upon Him, and by His stripes we are healed.

## January 2

**God wants you healed**. Jesus bore your sickness before He went to the cross. He was beaten, and with His stripes you were healed. He bore your sins on the cross.

Jesus has paid the price for every sickness you might suffer. He has paid the price for every sin you have committed, and every sin you will commit. This is hard to grasp, but the scriptures tell us that this is true.

Learn scriptures like these. Have them committed to your memory. A good way to do this is to write some basic healing scriptures on a piece of paper. The one below is a good one to do this with. Then post it on your refrigerator or bathroom mirror. Every time you see it, quote it out loud.

Learning to memorize scriptures is good. Quoting them daily is good. Reading them is good. Your ear hears when you quote them, your spirit hears, your mind is renewed. Seeing them is also important.

> 1 Peter 2:24 - who Himself bore our sins in His own body on the tree, that we, having died to sins, might live for righteousness—by whose stripes you were healed.

## January 3

**God wants you healed.** God set up blessings and curses in Deuteronomy 28. That is what that whole chapter is devoted to. In the curses, there are many types of sickness listed separately. In verse 61, it says any sickness or disease not listed, which means ALL sickness and diseases, are under the curse of the law.

The scripture below in the New Testament says that you are redeemed from the curse of the law. So, God set it up that you are completely redeemed from all sickness and all disease.

You have sickness thrown at you all the time. So many TV commercials are for medicines. You constantly have thoughts of sickness being put into your mind. When a lot of people get the flu, or some other disease, the news brings it to your attention.

Learn to ignore the commercials and the news. One minister said he used to always pray for the person in the commercials, and since they got well in the commercial, he got used to seeing people get well when he prayed for them.

Learn God wants you well. Learn to pray for others for healing. Don't ever stop.

> Galatians 3:13 - Christ has redeemed us from the curse of the law, having become a curse for us (for it is written, "Cursed is everyone who hangs on a tree"),

## January 4

**God wants you healed.** Nature cleans water by having it rush over rocks. As it moves along through streams it tumbles over rocks and slowly gets cleaned.

Man has introduced impurities which have stopped this purification for many areas around the world. Many soaps, cleansers, and also medications have caused the water to be polluted.

In the scripture below, it is talking about a man reading scriptures to his wife. The Word will sanctify her, it will cleanse her. This is washing her by the water of the Word. The Word is the Bible, it is scriptures.

If a woman is single, she can read the Bible herself. A man will also be cleansing himself as he reads the Bible out loud to his wife. The Word is like water to the body. It cleanses the body.

The word "sanctify" can also mean "to set apart." As you read the Word, it sets you apart from the world. It purifies you. For these actions to take place, you need to read the Word out loud for this cleansing.

As your body is cleansed, it is also being healed.

> Ephesians 5:26 - that he might sanctify and cleanse her with the washing of water by the Word.

## January 5

**God wants you healed.** The scripture below is one to use and to keep. It says, "For they…"; the word 'they' refers to scriptures, all scriptures, God's Word. Then it says that they are 'health' to all of their flesh. The Hebrew word used for health also means medicine.

When you read scriptures out loud, it is like you are taking medicine. It is best to use scriptures which will also renew your mind, and will feed your spirit. Then you are getting full benefit from the scripture.

God wants you healed so much that He supplied you with lots of medicine. That is a good way to look at what this scripture says. Make this one of the basic scriptures which you use on a regular basis.

You can use this scripture also as medicine to prevent sickness. That will help keep you healed. Learn more of what the Bible tells you about healing. Share with friends what you have learned.

> Proverbs 4:22 - For they are life to those who find them and health to all their flesh.

## January 6

**God wants you healed.** There are ways in the scriptures to obtain your healing. Using scripture is an excellent way. Find scriptures that tell you that God will heal you.

There are many scriptures which do this. If you look at different pages in this book, you will find every page has a different scripture on it. What do you do with these scriptures?

Select three to five scriptures to use. This is a good way to start. Find scriptures that minister to you. Scriptures which show you the way you want to be.

First pray them. Then meditate on them by speaking them out loud to yourself, every day. Picture yourself healed, every day.

If you are well, this is a good preventative way to stay well. More about this will follow.

How do we know this works? In the Bible there are many places that tell you this works. The scripture on this page tells you that this works. This is your proof, this is your confidence.

> John 16:24 - Until now you have asked nothing in My name. Ask, and you will receive, that your joy may be full.

## January 7

**God wants you healed**. He sent His Word. Jesus' name is called "The Word of God." Jesus has been sent. We know from previous pages there are scriptures that say by the stripes of Jesus you are healed.

From Psalms, we have another scripture which says a similar thing. The Word was sent, and you are healed. You are also delivered from destruction. Meditate on the scripture to help renew your mind and to feed your spirit.

God loves you very much. He loves you so much that He sent His Son to earth that you might be saved and have eternal life. That is almost beyond comprehension. Sometimes that scripture is taken lightly.

Use several of these scriptures which give you these promises. Write them out on a piece of paper and study them. Memorize them. There will be a day when you realize how glad you are that you did this.

> Psalm 107:20 - He sent His Word and healed them, and delivered them from their destructions.

By Patricia L. Whipp

## January 8

**Receive your healing**. There are several ways that healings can be done. Not all healings are received in the same manner. The gifts of the spirit tell us that there are gifts of healing. We know from scripture that many people set their faith (James 1:6) and, because of their faith, they received healing.

The gifts of the spirit also include miracles. Miracles and the gift of healings are a result of a minister praying for someone. Anyone can minister in these areas. It does not need to be an ordained minister. Many people are lay ministers.

Healings can be done simply by prayer, by applying your faith, and by taking authority over the enemy. When you read the gospels you see that Jesus used many methods of healing.

There is no pattern, no formula by which things must always be done. Following God, letting the Holy Spirit lead you is the best method.

> 1 Corinthians 12: 9-10
> 9 to another faith by the same Spirit, to another gifts of healings by the same Spirit,
> 10 to another the working of miracles, to another prophecy, to another discerning of spirits, to another different kinds of tongues, to another the interpretation of tongues.

## January 9

**Receive your healing.** You can always obtain healing by setting your faith. This is a sure way to obtain healing. Find scriptures which apply to what you want for your healing, pray them and believe. If you have someone else pray for you, or with you, that strengthens the prayer.

Ten men who were lepers called out to Jesus. The Bible does not say anything about their faith, but they were certainly looking to Jesus for their healing. He told them to go to the priest because, under the law, before Jesus was raised from the dead, only the priest could declare them clean.

Note: They were not instantly healed, but as they went they were healed. They took the steps of seeking Jesus and following His instructions. When you use your faith, that is exactly what you do.

> Luke 17:12-14
> 12 Then as He entered a certain village, there met Him ten men who were lepers, who stood afar off.
> 13 And they lifted up their voices and said, "Jesus, Master, have mercy on us!"
> 14 So when He saw them, He said to them, "Go, show yourselves to the priests." And so it was that as they went, they were cleansed.

## January 10

**Receive your healing.** The centurion came to ask Jesus to heal his servant. Jesus said He would come and heal the servant. The centurion answered and said, "Lord, I am not worthy that You should come under my roof. But only speak a word, and my servant will be healed.

"For I also am a man under authority, having soldiers under me. And I say to this one, 'Go,' and he goes; and to another, 'Come,' and he comes; and to my servant, 'Do this,' and he does it."

Do you have any concept of how powerful words are, especially when we speak scripture? Speaking scripture sets the angels in motion to fulfill what is spoken.

Some would respond, but that was Jesus. Jesus told us that we were to perform greater works than He performed.

To do this, you have to watch what you say at all times. As you start watching your words, expect to see more come to pass.

Matthew 8:7 - And Jesus said to him, "I will come and heal him."

Verses 8 and 9 are quoted in the text above.

## January 11

**Receive your healing.** There was a woman with the issue of blood who found Jesus, made her way to Him in a crowd, and was healed. This woman had spent all of her money on doctors. With her problem, she was not supposed to be in the city, but she had heard of Jesus, she risked getting caught. She made her way to Him.

It is obvious she had set her faith. She set the time, when she touched His garment was the time she set. Jesus did not know she was there, but He was aware of when she drew the healing anointing from Him.

This concept of setting a point of contact can be a good way to set your faith. Set your faith, believe, and at the point of contact, receive. Jesus said she was made whole by her faith.

> Matthew 9:21 - For she said to herself, "If only I may touch His garment, I shall be made well."

## January 12

**Receive your healing.** God is concerned about small things. You don't need to have a broken leg, or cancer, or other serious things. If you have an irritation on your skin, in your body somewhere, don't hesitate to seek God for healing.

Something as simple as not sleeping well, anything which is a concern to you, is something which God is available to assist you with.

Yes, there are far more serious things, but our God is big enough to handle the big things, and is interested in the small things. If you want prayer support, you can always ask the elders at your church to pray for you.

> James 5:14 - Is anyone among you sick? Let him call for the elders of the church, and let them pray over him, anointing him with oil in the name of the Lord.

## January 13

**Receive your healing**. How do you receive your healing? Say, "I receive" as you are prayed for. If you are praying for yourself, say, "I receive." Do not doubt, do not waiver, receive your healing.

I know of one lady, in a healing line, who had an open wound that was bleeding. When she was prayed for it dried up and closed up. She kept saying, "I don't believe it!" She continued to say that. The wound opened back up and started bleeding again!

The words of your mouth are very important. You start as soon as you are prayed for knowing that you are healed. How do you know it? Because the Bible says that you are healed.

Learn to start thanking God for your healing. Trust God, and know that the healing is yours.

Once again, do not doubt, do not waiver.

James 1:6 - But let him ask in faith, with no doubting, for he who doubts is like a wave of the sea driven and tossed by the wind.

## January 14

**Receive your healing**. You need to learn to receive your healing. Does your healing always manifest immediately? When you pray for finances, are they in your account immediately? When you pray for a car, do you receive it immediately?

Often, there is a period of time between prayer for anything, and the time it arrives. When a healing does not manifest right away, it can cause concern, that can lead to doubt. It can be affecting your work, your feelings, every area of your life. That has much to do with it.

As with any area of faith, know that the healing process has started when the prayer was made. Watch for any area of improvement, and look for other things to praise God over.

One person who was praying for a leg, said he praised God because both his arms didn't hurt. His head didn't hurt, etc.

> James 1:2-3
> 2 My brethren, count it all joy when you fall into various trials,
> 3 knowing that the testing of your faith produces patience.

## January 15

**Maintain your healing**. In order to maintain your healing, one of the first things you need to do is watch your mouth. Once you are prayed for, if your healing is not complete, it is started. Talk about it as completed.

If your healing has not started, you see no change, do not be moved by what you see. God's Word says that you should call those things which be not as though they were.

When you go to a doctor, do you see changes when you walk out of his office? Usually not. Whether you were prayed for, or you went to a doctor, you need to follow instructions.

Meditate on the scriptures used when you were healed. If none were used, pick healing scriptures that witness to you. Meditate on those.

Satan is a thief. He works on stealing the Word from Christians. He also steals healings when he can.

This is from the parable of sowing seeds. The seed is the Word of God.

> Mark 4:15 - And these are the ones by the wayside where the Word is sown. When they hear, Satan comes immediately and takes away the Word that was sown in their hearts.

## January 16

**Maintain your healing.** Have you noticed that scriptures are always included with the teachings? There is healing in scripture. There is power in scripture. Quoting scripture sends your angels to work.

Quoting scriptures is a part of warfare against Satan, who has caused your sickness. Learn to look for scriptures to use, learn to meditate scripture. Satan may attempt to bring your sickness back.

As a preventative, have at least one scripture which you quote daily to maintain your health. The following is not a healing scripture, it is here to show you what to do, and why do it.

There are scriptures in the New Testament which say the same thing. Do not think that this is just an Old Testament teaching.

This scripture may not use the word 'healing,' but good success includes the concept of healing.

> Joshua 1:8 - This Book of the Law shall not depart from your mouth, but you shall meditate in it day and night, that you may observe to do according to all that is written in it. For then you will make your way prosperous, and then you will have good success.

## January 17

**Maintain your healing.** You do have an enemy. This enemy would like to steal your healing. There are people who do not believe that. God has an enemy, so we have an enemy. His name is Satan. You have authority over him, you tell him to leave in the Name of Jesus, and he must do that.

He comes to steal the Word of God that you have in your heart. This is why it is so important to read the Bible every day, and to read scriptures out loud to yourself. You keep the Word alive and fresh in your spirit.

You have authority over the devil. You have the right to tell him to leave, and he has to. The problem is that he has a short attention span. He has to be told this again and again.

Don't quit. Don't give up. You have the victory. It has been promised to you. You have to hold onto the victory.

You stay focused on the Word so that you do not forget that you have the victory.

> Luke 8:11-12
> 11 "Now the parable is this: The seed is the Word of God.
> 12 Those by the wayside are the ones who hear; then the devil comes and takes away the Word out of their hearts, lest they should believe and be saved.

## January 18

**Maintain your healing.** Do you have doubts lurking in the back of your mind, very faintly? Maybe that a healing is not complete? Maybe it will return?

I know of one lady who had a miraculous healing. The doctor had told her the disease would return in ten years. She never told anyone who could have ministered to her about what the doctor had said, but the memory was alive in her mind.

In ten years, the disease returned with a vengeance. It came so fast, and so hard, that there was not time to counsel her and get her faith built up enough to recover. She died.

Any doubts in your mind about your healing must be dealt with and removed. When you are fully believing, when you know what the Bible says and that the Bible is true, then you have the victory.

If you have doubts, that is being double-minded. When you are double-minded, then you are unstable. Speak to doubts, tell them to leave.

Find healing scriptures that minister to you. Meditate on those. Read them out loud daily. Just keep them alive in your mind and spirit. Then you will keep those doubts out of your thoughts.

James 1:8 - a double-minded person is unstable in all his ways.

## January 19

**Maintain your healing.** You need to start controlling your thoughts! If you think of sickness, it will come out of your mouth. The scripture says, "…out of the abundance of the heart the mouth speaks." So if you dwell on something, if you keep thinking it, you will speak it.

If you keep talking sick, you will bring sickness on yourself. What do you do? First of all find a scripture. Psalm 107:2 says, "Let the redeemed of the Lord say so." You are redeemed, so say so. You are redeemed from sickness. Say so.

Next, paint a picture in your mind of how you want to see yourself. If you are not like you picture yourself, try to find a physical picture of yourself the way you want to see yourself. Keep that posted somewhere. Now "post" that picture in your mind.

Whenever your thoughts wander where they shouldn't be, pull up the scripture you are standing on, meditate that scripture. Pull up the mental image and view that.

> Luke 6:45 - A good man out of the good treasure of his heart brings forth good; and an evil man out of the evil treasure of his heart brings forth evil. For out of the abundance of the heart his mouth speaks.

## January 20

**Maintain your healing.** Is there any fear or doubt in your mind about your healing being real? This is not talking about how you feel, but how you think. Those fears must be dealt with. Your spirit needs to be fed scriptures so that you know that you know you are the healed. Your mind also needs to know that you are healed.

The fears and doubts are the same way, you need to tell those to leave you and be rid of them. This sounds like I am just being "pushy," but it is so real. The fears and doubts are not from God, and you don't want anything from Satan.

Normally, I would approach anything from the positive. Personally, I would meditate on healing scriptures. I would speak to the fear and doubts, tell them to leave me, and meditate on healing.

There is one time, years ago, when for one day I did meditate on fear scriptures, but I settled that in my mind and that is over. If you need to settle in your mind that fear is not of God, then do that. Get those thoughts out of your mind.

> Jeremiah 17:14 - Heal me, O LORD, and I shall be healed; save me, and I shall be saved, for You are my praise.

## January 21

**Maintain your healing.** It would be wonderful if all healings were instant. But they are not. That doesn't mean your body is not working! In fact, if you will check you may see some areas of improvement. Simply stand believing, because some things take more time.

Don't compare yourself to someone else; they received their healing of the same thing in two weeks, and you've gone four weeks. Your eyes are on worldly things, not God.

Stand, believing, and know that the Bible is true.

> Hebrews 6:11-12
> 11 And we desire that each one of you show the same diligence to the full assurance of hope until the end,
> 12 that you do not become sluggish, but imitate those who through faith and patience inherit the promises.

## January 22

**Walking in divine health.** The best way to learn to walk in divine health is to start before you get sick. Part of what was said in the maintaining your health pages definitely applies to walking in divine health.

You want to find scriptures, find several scriptures that minister to you. Scriptures that show God wants you healed, that show how you look healed. Read them out loud daily. This gives you your flu shot, daily. It actually gives you a total body shot, daily.

Memorizing the scriptures is great. What you want to do is get them fully into your spirit, and you want your mind totally renewed. Your mind needs to be renewed, and your spirit fed on a regular basis. This is not a once in a lifetime thing.

Memorizing them is fine. But you need to periodically read them. You need to keep them active in your mind. You do this by both reading and speaking them.

Here are some suggested scriptures:

Psalm 103:1-3
1 Bless the LORD, O my soul; and all that is within me, bless His holy name!
2 Bless the LORD, O my soul, and forget not all His benefits:
3 Who forgives all your iniquities, Who heals all your diseases,

## January 23

**Walking in divine health.** Learning to stay healthy is how you walk in divine health. This is the best way to live.

There are several things which you should do to accomplish this. One of the things is to maintain your peace and your joy. We see in the scripture below that the joy of the Lord is your strength.

You need strength to maintain your health. When you are weak and rundown, you are not healthy.

Learn to laugh. Laughing is good for you. It also helps you to maintain your joy. Watch good comedies. Sometimes the older ones are better.

Joy is a fruit of the spirit. This means that you can call it up. You can do this with peace and with joy. Pray for yourself, tell these fruits to come forth. You can do this in praying for others as well.

> Nehemiah 8:10 - Then he said to them, "Go your way, eat the fat, drink the sweet, and send portions to those for whom nothing is prepared; for this day is holy to our Lord. Do not sorrow, for the joy of the LORD is your strength."

## January 24

**Walking in divine health.** Once again, God has an enemy, so you have an enemy. He will try to steal the Word of God from you. That is all he can do, but this is the reason that it is so important to keep the Word fresh in your mind and in your spirit.

Do not let up on your confessions, your Bible reading, also church attendance as well as praise and worship. These all help keep you healthy.

Listen to teachings on a regular basis. You can do this at home on TV, on your computer, in your car using CDs, or mp3s. Today there are many ways to do this. It does help.

Even pastors must do these things. They need to be feeding on the Word, they need to be receiving teaching from others. If this is true for pastors, how much more for the rest of us?

> Proverbs 4:20 - My son, give atten-
> tion to my words; incline your ear
> to my sayings.

January 25

**Walking in divine health.** What do you do with doubts? Personally I speak to them. I tell them to go in the name of Jesus. You do not want to waver in your mind. In the gospels, several times Jesus marveled at their unbelief. Doubting is unbelief.

It is so easy to think things like, "This is not a disease. This is because I'm overweight, so it's my fault, so God won't heal this." Where does it say that? True, it is best to lose the weight, it is best to keep yourself in good condition.

God asked me that exact question one time. He said, "Where in my Word does it say that Galatians 3:13 is not true if you are overweight?" I did not answer. I realized that my thoughts had been wrong. The weight problem was not a gluttony issue, it was due to other causes.

Romans 3:3-4

3 For what if some did not believe? Will their unbelief make the faithfulness of God without effect? 4 Certainly not! Indeed, let God be true but every man a liar. As it is written: "That you may be justified in your words, and may overcome when you are judged."

## January 26

**Walking in divine health.** Scripture tells us that as a man thinks, so is he. (Proverbs 23:7) What you think on will probably come out of your mouth. We know that out of the abundance of the heart the mouth speaks. (Matthew 12:34)

With these scriptures, it seems obvious that we want our mind on the good, on what we want to see. Definitely not on the bad, definitely not on what we don't want to happen.

I used to think that I had no control over my thoughts. That is a lie from the devil. Scripture tells you to renew your mind. You need to start immediately. You do this with scriptures. Find a scripture that ministers to you. Every time you realize that you are not thinking on the good, pull up the scripture you have chosen, and start quoting it out loud to yourself. This can be very softly.

When I first started, it might be four hours before I realized my mind had wandered again. Now, it is much less time. If you are thinking about how you feel, about pain, speak to the pain, tell it to leave you in the name of Jesus, and start quoting a scripture. Don't buy the lie that nothing is happening, it is.

> Philippians 3:13 - Brethren, I do not count myself to have apprehended; but one thing I do, forgetting those things which are behind and reaching forward to those things which are ahead,

## January 27

**Walking in divine health.** Praise God for your healing. Once you have been prayed for, or you have prayed for your healing, move into praising God. Thank Him for your healing. Thank God for everything He has done for you. Praise God for all that is good.

What does this do? It has you talking with God in a positive way, not a negative way. It has your mind off the problem. It has you operating in joy, and the joy of the Lord is your strength.

There are times when healing takes time. That is true if you are on medicine from a doctor, that may be true if you are on scriptures, which are medicine. The body takes time to mend. It has the process of healing built in, but not all healing is done as a miracle.

The important thing is for you to remember that you are healed. Scripture says to call those things which be not as though they were. This is not lying, this is saying what the scripture says. The scriptures say that you are healed, so speak that. Keep the words of your mouth in line with scripture. As you do this, watch your body line up with the Word of God.

> Romans 4:17 - (as it is written, "I have made you a father of many nations") in the presence of Him whom he believed—God, who gives life to the dead and calls those things which do not exist as though they did;

## January 28

**Walking in divine health.** To learn to walk in divine health, you need to learn to be consistent. Use scriptures regularly to maintain your health. That should be true for every area of your life, not just your health. You will benefit from doing this.

As an example, take three to five healing scriptures that you like. Read them out loud to yourself. If you have a family, do this as a family, children as well.

Doing this for three weeks gets you started. Basically, this has been called a flu shot. But it is much more than a flu shot. Everything, all sicknesses the children bring home from school, everything has to flee.

After three weeks, seek God to see how often this should be done.

God will see what you are doing. God will see this as being faithful. You are faithful to use His Word. He is interested in faithfulness, He likes to see His children be consistent even in the little details of life.

> Psalm 101:6 - My eyes shall be on the faithful of the land, that they may dwell with me; he who walks in a perfect way, he shall serve me.

# January 29

Meditation comes from God. The Bible talks about meditation from the beginning. Bible meditation is not like some eastern methods.

The Word used in the Bible for meditation means to mutter, or you quote scripture over and over. This can be very softly. It must be spoken, but it doesn't need to be heard by others.

Another thing which you can do is visualize the desired result. Visualize the healing completed.

For everything, it is necessary to meditate on the Word of God. It is necessary to believe the Word of God. It is necessary to trust God, and what He says in His Word. The Word, the Bible is important.

Is it possible to get healed without using the Word? It is. It happens. I am not sure it is possible to walk in divine health without using the Word. I know that many people do not realize the importance of the Word.

Learn to believe the Word, to trust in the Word, to talk the Word, and to walk the Word.

> Psalm 19:14 - Let the words of my mouth and the meditation of my heart be acceptable in Your sight, O LORD, my strength and my Redeemer.

By Patricia L. Whipp

## January 30

God's Word is true. There may be some verses that are not true, but they accurately describe what happened, or what someone said, that does not line up with the Word. Some verses in Job fit this comment.

God's Word is healing for you. It is medicine to your body. God has provided healing through His Word. He wants you well. He wants you walking in divine health.

If you will learn to trust God, if you will spend time in the Word, if you will learn what the Bible says, what more can you ask for? God is your shield, He is your provider. He has blessings for you.

Learn to walk with God. You don't have to know everything in the Bible, as long as you are sincere, trusting God, He will guide you to the steps you need to take. He will help you to learn what you need at the time.

Praise God. Thank Him for His Word, thank Him for His goodness. Let God be your guide and your teacher.

> Proverbs 30:5 - Every Word of God
> is pure; He is a shield to those who
> put their trust in Him.

## January 31

There was a man who had a withered hand. What would cause a withered hand? It could be caused by many things, but arthritis is something that could cause a hand to look withered. No matter what caused the problem, Jesus gave His body for it to be healed.

In this scripture, Jesus is angry with the rabbis because they were more concerned with the Sabbath than they were in seeing a man be healed. They were more concerned with their rules than they were with a person.

Jesus wanted everyone healed. He would give His body for everyone else's body to be healed. His body was beaten, and with every stripe He suffered, Jesus paid for the healing of everyone alive since that day.

Don't get into condemnation over a thought. The enemy is Satan. He has you bound, He is the one you want to attack with the Word, for it is like a two-edged sword.

Your healing has been paid for. When needed, also pray for others to be healed.

> Mark 3:5 - And when He had looked around at them with anger, being grieved by the hardness of their hearts, He said to the man, "Stretch out your hand." And he stretched it out, and his hand was restored as whole as the other.

By Patricia L. Whipp

## February 1

God will supply you with food and water. (Philippians 4:19) You have to trust God. You have to believe Him. Many people today do not eat healthy, and do not drink enough water.

There is so much 'junk' food available. It suits our taste buds, and we don't realize that we are robbing our body today. One minister was talking about 'diet soft drinks,' he felt they supplied his need for water.

I heard of one lady who lived for years on a type of cake produced as a snack food. Fortunately, she has been redeemed from this. Her family prayed, sought prayer from others, and she learned a better way to live.

Some people are so into 'health' that they have a fear of these types of food. You don't have to walk in fear, and you don't have to refuse to eat anything that is classified 'junk.'

Learn to seek God. Ask Him what is OK for you to do. You can find all sorts of contradictory information on the internet. Learn to use common sense, and let the Holy Spirit lead you in what is safe for you to do.

> John 6:35 - And Jesus said to them, "I am the bread of life. He who comes to Me shall never hunger, and he who believes in Me shall never thirst.

## February 2

God is always willing to heal people. The Israelites, when they had strayed from God, the day came that they wanted to repent, they wanted to return to God. They knew He would accept them, and they knew He would heal them. They knew His nature.

If you have strayed, or are praying for someone who has strayed from God, do not be concerned. God is quick to forgive once you confess what you have done. God is also quick to heal.

It is in the nature of God to want man to be whole, healed, and doing good. God is good and He wants nothing but the best for man. Sickness is not the best! God never makes someone sick, or wants anyone to be sick.

God does take advantage of your attention and teach you at times when you are sick, but He would do the same thing when you are well if you would give Him your attention. Keep that in mind as you learn to walk healed. Seek God, give Him your attention.

> Hosea 6:1 - Come, and let us return to the LORD; for He has torn, but He will heal us; He has stricken, but He will bind us up.

## February 3

Learn to walk in peace. Peace in itself is healing to your body. Doctors will tell you this. When you are not in peace, you are anxious, stressed, or some other condition which adds to your physical destruction.

God has given you peace. Jesus gave you His peace. Peace is yours. Many people want peace, but have no idea how to walk in peace. Learning what the scriptures say, and learning to love the scriptures, is a good step toward walking in peace.

Have you noticed that many doctors do not agree on some things? For example, they will differ on what foods are good for your body. Science is learning more every day about the body, but so far no one can put all of this together. One person was commenting to me today that she had an appointment with an expert on the subject she needs help with. The expert's response, "We don't know."

There is One who does know. That is the creator. God knows what your body needs at any given time. Step one, peace. You need to get quiet to hear for help on what you should do.

Spend time in the scriptures, develop a love for the scriptures.

> Psalm 119:165 - Great peace have those who love Your law, and nothing causes them to stumble.

## February 4

Your words have a lot to do with your health. If you speak negative words, your health will probably not be as good as it could be. It is very important to know what the Bible has to say about your health, and to speak those words.

Be aware, the Bible is truth. What happens, what we experience are facts. Learn to speak only the truth. If you keep speaking facts, you will keep experiencing them. For example, "Every winter I get the flu."

Am I suggesting that you lie? No, I am suggesting that you speak the truth, and let it cause the facts to line up with what you experience.

I read in a book to pray for people. The suggestion was made, if someone has a headache offer to pray for them. I had so many headaches that I was on headache medication, so that caught my attention. I realized God will heal headaches. I have not had a headache since then.

This had nothing to do with faith teaching, it wasn't a decision that I was aware of. It was as if I realized that I didn't have to have them. Forty years later, I have had opportunities to have a headache, but I refuse them.

> Proverbs 6:2 - You are snared by the words of your mouth; you are taken by the words of your mouth.

## February 5

God promises to answer prayer. If you pray in faith, He never says, "No." He doesn't even hear your prayer if you don't pray in faith. This does not mean that the prayers are instantly answered, but you are promised to receive them.

God wants you healed. He had His Son, Jesus, hung on a cross for you. Before Jesus was hung, He was beaten. With every strike of the whip, you were healed. Would God pay a price like that, and not want you healed?

This means that we just have to believe. There is no disease, no sickness, nothing, that cannot be healed. God also has spare parts for you; a new knee, a new hip, a new leg. God also uses doctors—eye surgeries, joint replacement surgeries are some areas that people are developing.

So, with all of these available, your faith should be very high. One thing I have found, don't tell God how to do it. Don't tell Him, I only want a new knee from you. Pray for a new knee, and let God decide how it is to be done. Be obedient if He sends you to a doctor, a healing meeting, a friend, or a prayer closet. He may do it in your sleep tonight.

> Mark 11:24 - Therefore I say to you, whatever things you ask when you pray, believe that you receive them, and you will have them.

## February 6

Have you ever seen a chicken, or duck, gather up their babies on their back? I watched a video of a duck gathering ducklings. It looked like that many babies could not possibly fit under her wings, but they did.

God wants you in the shadow of His wings. He wants you under His wings. He wants to protect you, to guide you, to let the calamities pass by.

Does this sound like God could possibly want you sick? No, God does not want you sick. Could He be teaching you something by your being sick? Yes, He does teach you something, but that is because He has your attention, not because that is the way He wants to teach you.

God loves you, He will never make you sick. He will never cause a sickness to come so that He can teach you or discipline you.

Learn to trust God, to follow His directions. He can warn you, and guide you, around problems and sickness. Make Him your refuge.

> Psalm 57:1 - Be merciful to me, O God, be merciful to me! For my soul trusts in You; and in the shadow of Your wings I will make my refuge, until these calamities have passed by.

## February 7

Healing is something that everyone needs at one time or another. We have covered four areas of healing: God wants you healed; how to receive your healing; how to maintain your healing; and walking in divine health.

There are steps that you need to take. This verse is not just for healing, but we are applying it to healing. Divine health is like the PhD of healing. Praise God for divine health.

So how do you get there? You learn to trust God. You learn what the Bible says about healing. You learn to apply scriptures as they are needed. You learn to not just walk in divine health for yourself, but to pray for others, and assist them to learn what you have learned.

Set this as the year that you are going to grow in the area of healing. Pray for others, walk in health for yourself. What do you do if you find yourself with a common cold? You take your authority and get rid of it.

Be diligent, learn scriptures, share with others, and walk in the light of the Word. Let your light shine so that others may see it and learn from you. (Matthew 5:16)

> 2 Timothy 2:15 - Be diligent to present yourself approved to God, a worker who does not need to be ashamed, rightly dividing the word of truth.

## February 8

God wants you well rested. That is essential to your health. You have choices to make. You can do an all work no play lifestyle. That is not God's design for your life, and does not make for a healthy life.

On the other side of the coin, you can do an all play no work. That is not good either. God expects you to do things for Him. What is fun for some people is work to others.

God wants you to have time to rest, He wants you to be in nice places. A quiet pasture with still waters is very peaceful.

Learn to have the quiet times in your schedule. God says one day a week. I know people who go weeks with no rest, then want to rest for several days.

Start by getting some rest in your life style. Then as you learn to hear God, and to know what He expects from you, let God lead you to what is right for you.

Praise God for green pastures and still waters.

Psalm 23:1-2
1 The LORD is my shepherd; I shall not want.
2 He makes me to lie down in green pastures; He leads me beside the still waters.

## February 9

God wants you well. If people try to tell you something different, remind them that their body is the temple of the Holy Spirit. He lives in you. He is there to teach, guide, and comfort you.

Think about that. Would God want to live in a sick temple? That makes no sense. God likes the best things. Why would He delay a healing, or in any way cause a sickness to be in your body?

People usually use this verse to tell you that it is your job to eat right, to only eat whatever types of food they consider the best, be sure you get plenty of rest, and don't abuse your body with drugs of any kind.

That is all good. But when people say that God delayed healing a sickness to teach them something, stop and think; would the Holy Spirit want to live in a sick body while He is teaching you something?

Trust God, and know that He wants the best for you.

> 1 Corinthians 6:19 - Or do you not know that your body is the temple of the Holy Spirit who is in you, whom you have from God, and you are not your own?

## February 10

God planned you from the beginning of time. You were no surprise to God, God wants you. If you were born with birth defects, that was not in God's plan. That was caused by the fall of man when Adam ate the forbidden fruit.

People who were born deformed, or with other birth defects, need to know that was not God's design for their life. They also need to know that God is a miracle working God. Believing for their total restoration is right. God did not design them that way. People who had something happen after they were born which has left them with a problem, that is also not God's plan, and it is not His design.

We have seen many people who have overcome amazing difficulties and done wonderful things. I am sure God has helped them to accomplish what they have done. Don't let that stop you from believing for God's best.

God's best is total restoration. There is no reason not to pray for a complete healing. Learning to do what you can and witnessing to people about what you accomplish is great. God helps you to make those accomplishments. Recognize that God did not make you handicapped, and that was not for His purpose.

> Psalm 139:14 - I will praise You, for I am fearfully and wonderfully made; marvelous are Your works, and that my soul knows very well.

By Patricia L. Whipp

## February 11

Don't always be looking ahead. What is going to happen tomorrow? You need to concentrate on today. Also, you need to remember where you came from, Who created man, how He designed you.

God formed man from the dust of the earth. He made the female from the male. So we all come from the dust of the earth. He created man perfect. He created your bodies to last, He created you to be healthy.

Don't ever forget where you came from. Sickness and disease were not a part of God's plan for your life. He wanted man to be healthy, alive, alert, full of energy. He wanted man to enjoy the earth, and the things He provided for them.

The Bible is a product of God's works. It is also given to us for our understanding and help. Learn to study the Bible. Learn to meditate on all of God's works; the planets, the earth, the sky, and the Bible.

Find scriptures that promise healing in the Bible. Meditate on those, as well as other scriptures. Maintaining your health, or becoming healthy, are all included in the Bible.

Psalm 143:5 - I remember the days of old; I meditate on all Your works; I muse on the work of Your hands.

# February 12

God's way is perfect. His Word is pure. We know that the scriptures are medicine for us. There is healing of flesh, the body, the soul including renewing of the mind, and refueling for the spirit.

Learn to use the Word of God for healing. There are times when it may be necessary to take medication made by man. It just happens. I recently had a surgery, and I have been very glad for medication.

But, take all medication with scripture. The scripture will work on you, and can purify the medicine you are taking. Do not feel that things need to be one or the other. God does use doctors. There are also doctors who use scripture.

Guidance is helpful. You don't always go to a Christian doctor, just as you do not always go to a Christian mechanic. Let God lead you.

Learn to be led, to trust God. You may be a witness to the non-Christian worker. You may water some seed that has been sown.

Always use the Word. Know that scriptures are pure and trust God for the results.

> 2 Samuel 22:31 - As for God, His way is perfect; the Word of the LORD is proven; He is a shield to all who trust in Him.

## February 13

The words of your mouth are important. I have heard children being taught that "words" are just sounds. How sad. Words are very important. So few people today have any idea of the importance of words.

Just as true are instructions from the Lord. Many people think that what is meant is when you hear God correct you. That is true, but what is not understood is that it can very easily be correction when you hear a Bible verse you had never heard, or not understood before.

If you hear a minister preach something, and you see it in the Bible, then you know it is there. If you have not been doing what that scripture says to do, your conscience should alert you. That is God, as much as if He spoke to you.

If you are reading the Bible, you might see something you hadn't realized before, such as the importance of forgiving others. If you didn't know this, and you read that verse, when you recognize what it says, that is a correction.

Now, it is life to you to follow the instruction. Life means health is included. It is health to you to follow the instructions in the Bible. Read your Bible.

> Proverbs 10:17 - He who keeps instruction is in the way of life, but he who refuses correction goes astray.

## February 14

God is love. God loves you so much that He gave His only begotten Son for you. God gave Jesus for you personally. God also loves you as much as He loves Jesus. Think about those things.

Jesus went to the cross for you because He loves you. Jesus paid the price for your salvation. That salvation includes your healing. Any sickness, any disease, any physical problem you might have, Jesus has paid the price for it.

When sickness, diseases, anything comes on you, remember that the price has been paid. You have the right to demand good health, because you have authority over all power of the enemy.

Choose to walk in divine health. Line your confession up with your prayers. Start choosing to bypass all sickness that attempts to come on you. Don't give in to sickness or disease.

As you make this decision, you will find less opportunities for sickness coming your way. Praise God for good health.

> John 3:16 - For God so loved the world that He gave His only begotten Son, that whoever believes in Him should not perish but have everlasting life.

By Patricia L. Whipp

## February 15

Do you know someone who is having mental problems? This could even be a child, it could be autism. It could also be a senior who is starting to forget things. It could be you. Are you so busy, so confused with news reports contrary to the Bible, that you don't know how to handle it?

We have the mind of Christ. "I have the mind of Christ." Make that a part of your daily confession if you feel that you need it. God wants your mind healthy as well as your body. The mind is a part of the soul, God wants your spirit, soul, and body all to be healthy.

You can pray any scripture, including the one below, over yourself or anyone else that you are praying for. ADHD and ADD are both problems frequently diagnosed today. Pray this over people with either of these disorders.

As with anything, don't be moved by what you see. Only be moved by what God tells you, and God speaks to you through His Word, through scriptures.

> 1 Corinthians 2:16 - For "who has known the mind of the LORD that he may instruct Him?" But we have the mind of Christ.

## February 16

When people have a disease that is considered deadly, especially when they have been told they only have a limited time to live, it is very easy to step into fear. Fear alone is deadly. You need to eliminate fear from your life. Fear is the opposite of faith.

Something to help you put things in a good perspective is to realize that to be absent from the body is to be present with the Lord. Death has no hold on a Christian. It just means you change locations of where you live.

However, there is no disease which God cannot heal. For some people, they may not have their faith built up enough to handle some things. This is why I stress learning to walk in divine health. Build up your faith, for yourself and to pray for others.

Notice also, in the scripture below, what God has given you. He has given you power, love, and a sound mind. God has given those to you, protect them.

Praise God, thank Him for what He has given you. Exercise your faith that it may grow. He has given you a spirit of power, of love and a sound mind. Thank you, Jesus.

> 2 Timothy 1:7 - For God has not given us a spirit of fear, but of power and of love and of a sound mind.

By Patricia L. Whipp

## February 17

Your bones are very important. You want healthy bones. You want to do what you can to maintain healthy bones. Keep yourself joyful. Laugh a lot, joy is very important to your health.

One translation says doom and gloom dry up the bones. That makes sense. Have you ever been around someone who always sees the bad side of things? They are always complaining, looking at everything that can go wrong.

That kind of an attitude is very bad on your health. But joy, laughter, loving life is like a medicine. We know that scriptures are medicine to your body, but this is like a medicine to your bones.

Find funny movies, some of the old ones are the best. Several years ago, I was given DVDs of old Carol Burnett shows. There are some funny scenes in there.

Science has also verified that doom and gloom attitudes are bad for your health. God told us that years ago, but science has proven it is true.

Spending time in praise and worship is also good. If you have never been drunk in the spirit, it is very good. There are no bad effects either.

Proverbs 17:22 - A merry heart does good, like medicine, but a broken spirit dries the bones.

## February 18

Are you in need of strength? Hannah, Samuel's mother, prayed for strength; she prayed for the bows of the wicked to be broken, and for strength for the one's who had stumbled. Have you been weak, stumbled and need strength?

Hannah's prayer was answered, you can use this for strength. Have you stumbled? Use this prayer for strength and for your legs to be strong and for no more stumbling. Hold the picture in your mind of no more stumbling.

The joy of the Lord is your strength. Learn to walk with God in His joy. (Nehemiah 10:17) Walking in joy, dancing in joy, is a way to increase your strength.

Meditating on scriptures strengthens your faith, and gives you a picture of your health being good. Maintain the picture of your legs functioning perfectly, maintain the picture of being strengthened.

Praise God for His healing that He gives. Praise Him for good health.

> 1 Samuel 2:4 - "The bows of the mighty men are broken, and those who stumbled are girded with strength.

## February 19

What is truth?  The Bible is truth.  Several scriptures  tell you this. You do need to understand that some scriptures are simply quoting what a person said.  They are not truth.  The scriptures of what God has said are truth.

Facts are what we see in this world.  They are often distorted.  We see popular people doing things that God said not to do, and some are earning good money for doing things that seem wrong.

A doctor's report is based on facts.  The Bible says that Jesus paid the price for our healing.  There are many places where the scriptures tell us that by the stripes of Jesus we are healed.  This is where you need to decide whose report will you believe.

You have a choice.  You are going to walk the world's way, or God's way.  I can tell you that God's way is life.  It will be life while you are in the world, and it will be life in heaven when you graduate from this world. (Deuteronomy 30:19)

This is an area that some people have a problem, but if you will line up your report, what you say, with God and the Bible, then you will walk and talk by faith; not by what you see, not by what the doctor says.

The choice is yours; God says, chose life.

2 Corinthians 5:7 - For we walk by faith, not by sight.

## February 20

Have you noticed that I frequently use scriptures? In praying for healing, I frequently use scriptures. In the scripture below, this is talking about how Jesus is preparing His church, how He is cleansing His bride.

This is an example for husbands of what they should do for their wives, but it is talking about Christ and the church. (Ephesians 5:26) The word sanctify can mean to cleanse, to heal, to purify. One example said to cleanse a leper of leprosy. That is a healing.

When we meditate scripture, read scripture out loud to ourselves, we are allowing Jesus to cleanse us. This is how spots and wrinkles can be removed. Jesus is coming for a church without spot or wrinkle.

Are people healed without reading scripture? Yes, they are, people who are not born again are healed. That is done as a sign and a wonder for the non-Christian. The Christian, especially one who has been walking in this for years, is expected to grow.

Read your Bible, meditate on scriptures, trust God, and receive your healings.

> John 6:63 - It is the Spirit who gives life; the flesh profits nothing. The words that I speak to you are spirit, and they are life.

## February 21

Do you know anyone whom the doctors have told them they have a terminal disease? What does the Bible say about this? The Bible says that they have every right to be free from that disease.

Has the person decided they will not accept the doctor's report? Have they prayed, or been prayed for, and accepted the report of the Bible? Then the person needs to be standing on scriptures. Quoting those scriptures daily.

"I shall not die, but live, and declare the works of the Lord." That is the scripture for today. That is an excellent verse for someone to use. I always suggest that more than one scripture is used, but this is one of those that builds a picture in their mind.

Actually, anyone can declare the works of the Lord. It can be done immediately, as the healing is being completed. This time is a good time to meditate scripture.

What can stop the healing? One thing is time. If a person is bleeding to death, there may not be time to save them. Don't procrastinate in making a decision. Believe and receive quickly.

> Psalm 118:17 - I shall not die, but live, and declare the works of the LORD.

## February 22

Are you a Christian? Have you made Jesus your Lord and Savior? This actually puts you in a different group of people than those that are in the world. It puts your home in heaven, and puts you on earth on assignment.

Jesus died on a cross; by accepting Him, it is as if you were crucified on that cross also. But, before the cross, He suffered, He was beaten. By those stripes, He bore every sickness and every disease that the devil will try to put on you. The price for every healing you need has been paid. Satan has no right to put those on you.

This is where we need to walk. Don't accept anything when symptoms come. Let the devil know that he has no right to put that on you. Walk free, knowing that those symptoms do not belong there and they have to leave.

This is walking in divine health. There are times when you will have to exercise your authority. Using scripture to maintain divine health is always wisdom.

Praise God, thank Him for the price that has been paid for you, and walk in the blessings.

> Galatians 2:20 - I have been crucified with Christ; it is no longer I who live, but Christ lives in me; and the life which I now live in the flesh I live by faith in the Son of God, who loved me and gave Himself for me.

## February 23

Often prayer is being asked by someone who is a Christian, knows what the Bible says, and has been doing "all the right things." They pray, have friends in agreement with them, quote their Bible verses out loud several times a day.

This Psalm says that God will not withhold from anyone who walks uprightly. Don't let the enemy lie to you. Don't start thinking, "I did this wrong yesterday. I yelled at John today," etc. Do not get into doubt and unbelief over things.

Uprightly can be achieved quickly. When you yelled at John, did you apologize? If not, do so now. Confess your sins, not to man, to God. Take communion, this can be done by yourself, at home. You are then walking uprightly again.

David was a man who knew the power of God's forgiveness. David messed up big time. When he realized what he had done, he asked God for forgiveness. God forgave him.

You can always get straight with God. Then you know that He will withhold nothing good.

Healing is His will and it is good.

Psalm 84:11 - For the LORD God is a sun and shield; the LORD will give grace and glory; no good thing will He withhold from those who walk uprightly.

## February 24

What is very important when you pray for anything is to hold fast to your confession of hope, without wavering.

Doctor's reports often cause doubt and unbelief. If you accept these reports, then your confession of faith wavers.

This is important in praying for healing as well as other things. Do not yield. What the Bible says is true. Do not ever forget that. The doctor's reports simply tell you what you need to take authority over.

Decide today. Are you going to believe the reports of others, or are you going to believe the Word of God? It all starts with a decision. Don't yield, don't sway. Make your decision, and stick to it.

Don't ask why someone didn't get healed. Just watch your mouth, your confession, and what you do. Don't let your faith waver, don't become double-minded. Hold fast to your confession. That is your hope.

God is faithful. God never wavers. Praise God, thank Him for your healing.

> Hebrews 10:23 - Let us hold fast the confession of our hope without wavering, for He who promised is faithful.

## February 25

Do you feel odd about going out, praying for people, getting them healed, and talking about the kingdom of God? Do you feel that was for the disciples, and you are not a disciple? After sending the twelve out, Jesus sent seventy.

Who were these seventy? They must have been people who followed Him. They must have been people who listened to Him. We know they did not have the privileges that the twelve had, there were times when He explained things just to the twelve.

What happened to the seventy? They came back and were very excited. They had the same experiences that the twelve had. The demons left, the sick were healed. They found that they could do the same things the others had done.

There were about a hundred and twenty in the upper room. So there were more than the seventy plus the twelve disciples.

This should prove to you that you have the same rights that the twelve had. You can pray for the sick, you can speak to devils in the name of Jesus, and you can tell people about the kingdom of God.

> Luke 10:9 - And heal the sick there, and say to them, 'The kingdom of God has come near to you.'

## February 26

An area that is not often applied in healing is your authority. You have authority over all works of darkness. You do not have authority over people or property that is not yours, or land, cities, etc. where you own no property.

If someone asks for prayer for healing, they have given you the right to use your authority. Would anyone want to stay sick? Sometimes the answer to that is yes. They like the pain medication they are on, they like the attention that they receive.

Certainly for yourself you have authority. For a child where you have a responsibility, who has not developed enough to be responsible for themselves, a child that because of mental problems cannot be responsible for themselves, you have the right to use your authority.

Using your authority on yourself is very good. It works well on any pain you have as well. This is an area where you can use your faith. Develop your faith in your authority over your health.

> Matthew 16:19 - And I will give you the keys of the kingdom of heaven, and whatever you bind on earth will be bound in heaven, and whatever you loose on earth will be loosed in heaven."

## February 27

There are many ways to be healed. There is not just one way, God does not have a favorite way. God likes variety. That is why there are so many different flowers, birds, butterflies, and on and on.

There are some people that think we always need to anoint with oil when praying for the sick; there are people that think we should always use our authority; another is to always pray in agreement.

In the verse below, it says that the prayer of faith will save the sick. This is also translated will heal you, or make you well. The verse before this is talking about anointing with oil, the verse after is talking about confessing your sins.

If you have come to the elders for healing, they may anoint you with oil, they will pray for you and the prayer of faith will heal you. If you have sinned, you may come to the elders, confess your sin, and be set free.

Once again, there is no one way to do this. There are many ways to receive healing. God wants you healed. The best way is to follow the leading of the Holy Spirit.

> James 5:15 - And the prayer of faith will save the sick, and the Lord will raise him up. And if he has committed sins, he will be forgiven.

## February 28

Starting possibly in the 19th century, and hopefully increasing even more now in the 21st century, there are those who are growing their faith.

In Luke, there is a story of a woman who goes to an unjust judge. She is so persistent that the judge gives her what she is asking for simply because of her persistence, not for any other reason.

The verse below is in red. Jesus asked, when He returns will he really find faith on the earth? In seeking your healing, let Jesus find faith. Some versions add the word persistent; will He really find persistent faith on the earth?

Certainly healing is one area that there should be persistent faith. It is promised to us. I know of people who have given up, or given in. Don't be one of these. If you are standing for several things, you might want to get one healing, then another. But, don't quit.

Jesus died for your healing, He bore stripes for your healing. Know that healing is yours, let the enemy know that healing is yours, receive your healing, and be persistent.

> Luke 18:8 - I tell you that He will avenge them speedily. Nevertheless, when the Son of Man comes, will He really find faith on the earth?"

## February 29

Do you, or someone you know, have problems breathing, possibly even having to use an oxygen tank? God can heal that problem. There is no sickness or disease that cannot be healed by God. He wants you well.

As with any healing, using scriptures is always good. There are also general scriptures that tell you that God heals. In part, you are renewing your mind, and you are refreshing your spirit in many areas. So scriptures showing you what you want healed are good.

When you are healed, you need to use scriptures to walk in divine health. That is not only maintaining the healings you have received, but it is seeing to it that other things do not come on you.

When God formed Adam, He breathed into Adam's nostrils with the breath of life. Maintaining a picture of that can help your mind seeing God doing and maintaining your breathing. That scripture is here to use for your breathing.

> Genesis 2:7 - And the LORD God formed man of the dust of the ground, and breathed into his nostrils the breath of life; and man became a living being.

## March 1

Are you praying for a child? Do you or your spouse seem to be unable to have a child, or have the doctors told you that you cannot have a child? There are many examples in the Bible of women who could not have a child.

Hannah wanted a child, she prayed, and God blessed her with a child. Sarah was past the age of child bearing, when God blessed her and Abraham with Issac. In the New Testament, Elizabeth became pregnant with John the Baptist when she was reaching old age.

I have a friend who the doctors told there was no way she could have a child. Her husband laid hands on her, prayed for a child, and she became pregnant. God still does miracles today, not just in Bible days.

If you are in this situation, take scriptures, meditate on them, pray, trust God. As with anything you are praying for, continue meditating on scriptures. These build the truth into your mind and your spirit. Believe and receive.

> Deuteronomy 7:14 - You shall be blessed above all peoples; there shall not be a male or female barren among you or among your livestock.

## March 2

God placed you on this earth, received you as His child when you became born again, and has made everything you would need in this life available for you. God does not do things part way. He makes provision for you.

Health is a part of what is needed for your life. God has made health available to you. There is an enemy who is attempting to see to it that you do not have the things you need, including health. But you have authority over that enemy.

Don't ever doubt that God wants you well. Don't ever think that healing is not available. If you have found yourself angry with God, He is not upset over that. It does hinder your healing. So repent, forgive yourself, and go forward.

Notice, these things are available through the knowledge of God. Learn what is available to you, study your Bible.

Praise God for all things that pertain to life and godliness. Receive what God has given to you.

> 2 Peter 1:3 - as His divine power has given to us all things that pertain to life and godliness, through the knowledge of Him who called us by glory and virtue,

## March 3

God has always wanted His people healed. There has always been provision made for healing. I have heard preachers say differently, but read your Bible. You can find provisions made throughout the Old Testament.

After both David and his son Solomon died, there were many kings. Many were very bad, and there were also very good kings. Hezekiah was a good king. We see below that God healed the people at Hezekiah's request.

When Moses led the people out of Egypt, God healed the people. The morning when they left, there was not one feeble person among them. With that many people, who were poorly treated, poorly fed, and even many elderly, there had to be sickness. God healed them after the passover. None were feeble. (Psalm 105:37)

Can't you see, as a son (or daughter) of God, that He wants you well? He wants His people healed. He wants no sickness or disease among His people.

Never doubt the willingness of God to heal you. No matter what you have done, or how you have treated God, He wants you healed. He loves you, He sent Jesus to the cross for you, He wants you healed.

> 2 Chronicles 30:20 - And the LORD listened to Hezekiah and healed the people.

By Patricia L. Whipp

## March 4

What is your soul? It is your mind, your emotions, and your will. All sickness is not physical. If your emotions are bad, it can cause stress, anxiety, fear, frustration, and other things, all of which can lead to sickness. Negative emotions can lead to physical illness.

Mental disorders are also a form of sickness. This sounds like you do not want problems with your soul. Keeping your soul healthy is a big step to keeping both you and your body healthy.

Most people do not realize how many problems you can cause with your mouth. Saying things like, "That scared me to death." "The pain in my foot is killing me." Do you really want to die early? Not many people want to. Don't keep talking death.

"I caught a cold." Why did you catch it? At the point this statement is said, it might have been a sneeze, or a sniffle. Tell the cold to keep going, tell it that it can't stay in your body.

Use your tongue to praise God. Use it to witness the love and goodness of God to others. Do not use it to make foolish comments.

> Proverbs 21:23 - Whoever guards his mouth and tongue keeps his soul from troubles.

## March 5

God never changes. He has made promises to His children. You have the promises He made to all before you, as well as the promises He has made to Christians. You are released from all of the curses, all of the problems.

God loves us so much that He will forgive and forget, the minute you repent. As we see from David and others, God has always been one to forgive once someone repents.

God has made healing available today for everyone. The heathen are healed as well as the Christian. You have the right to walk healed by using your authority. If your faith needs a boost, you can have prayer from others.

The Jews had healing available, but it did require going to a priest. From the records written and the Jewish history, that might not have been exercised frequently.

Today, this century, there are healing revivals going on around the world. Don't miss out, receive healing, pray for others, witness to people about a God who is good, loves you and wants the best for you.

> 1 Samuel 15:29 - And also the Strength of Israel will not lie nor relent. For He is not a man, that He should relent."

## March 6

Do you have friends, children, or other people you know who have backslidden? Maybe you have backslidden from God. Spiritually, there is a healing needed. God is concerned about healing those relationships.

God wants you healed, spirit, soul, and body. God wants everyone healed, in every area of their life. This is something very few people understand. It's not just the physical body that God looks over. Areas of the soul and of the spirit are just as important to God.

When someone is backslidden, their mind is not renewed to God, and the spirit can become endangered. The mind needs scriptures to keep it renewed, the spirit feeds on scriptures. Scriptures are medicine to the body. They renew the mind. Sounds like they are a type of medicine to the mind.

Keep yourself healthy with the Word of God. Read the Word daily. Meditate the Word. Listen to teachings.

> Jeremiah 3:22 - "Return, you back-sliding children, and I will heal your backslidings." "Indeed we do come to You, for You are the LORD our God.

## March 7

Are you, or someone you pray for, in pain? Is there a disease that is causing you problems, pain, discomfort? God is a healing God. God never changes. David called out to God when he was distressed, and God did miracles for David.

God never changes. He is the same yesterday, today, and tomorrow. If you call out to God, He will help you. The devil is the one who wants you sick. He is the one who does all he can to keep you that way.

Trust God. Believe God for your healing. Speak to the pain to stop. Jesus not only bore your sickness when He was beaten, He bore your pain. Is there a question about what is causing the pain? If so, seek God to find the cause. If not, stand strong on your authority over pain.

If you have already prayed, then receive prayers in agreement from others. Read your Bible. Pick scriptures that you will read out loud. Trust God and know that He will never fail you.

> 2 Samuel 22:7 - In my distress I called upon the LORD, and cried out to my God; He heard my voice from His temple, and my cry entered His ears.

## March 8

If you have been given a report from a doctor that is very negative, it can feel like a shadow of death. If the report says you will die in one day, or maybe within a few years, it can feel like a shadow of death.

Praise God, that is the best the doctor knows. But there is a God in heaven who heals. There is a God who wants you healed. He has a totally different report for you. His report is health and life.

God is always with you to comfort you, to protect you, to guide you. Draw from God, use His wisdom, follow His plans. This means you need to read and study the Bible. That is the only way to learn what He has for you. In the Bible is life, light, and wisdom.

You need to find scriptures that paint a picture of you healed, healthy, and going forward. If possible have agreement on your prayer. Then meditate on those scriptures, and watch them come to pass in your life.

> Psalm 23:4 - Yea, though I walk through the valley of the shadow of death, I will fear no evil; for You are with me; Your rod and Your staff, they comfort me.

## March 9

God is good. He wants you walking in His goodness. Goodness includes good health. Sickness is not good! Sickness was not a part of God's creation. When iniquity was found in the devil, that is when bad things were formed.

All sickness and disease are from the devil. A Christian has authority over these things. God has given you good things. Walk with God. His desire is for goodness and mercy to follow you all the days of your life.

Many people have a wrong concept of what God wants for them. They also have a wrong concept of where all bad things came from. Learn the truth. Tell others what God's desire is for them.

When your life is ended, and you go to heaven, then you will dwell in the house of the Lord forever. We know that you will have your own mansion. Build this picture into you. Build the knowledge that God is good into you. Know what is evil, know that you have authority over all evil.

> Psalm 23:6 - Surely goodness and mercy shall follow me all the days of my life; and I will dwell in the house of the LORD forever.

By Patricia L. Whipp

## March 10

Many born-again Christians say that they don't hear God. They also imply that they do not know how to know what God's will is on a matter. First, read your Bible.

The Jews had scrolls that they had God's Word on. Even for the Old Testament, they were told if they would seek God with all of their heart and all of their soul, that they would find Him. Your soul is your mind, emotions and will.

God will not force Himself on you. If you are seeking healing, that is no different than anything else. What is different is that Christians can pray for anyone and they are often healed.

God wants you healed. As you become more mature, you are expected to use your faith. There comes a day when you must grow up. The Holy Spirit is your teacher. He will teach you things. You must take steps. He is a gentleman. He doesn't force knowledge on you.

Healing is available. God wants you healed. Seek God, seek Him through ministers that believe the whole Bible. Also, read the Bible. Pray, ask the Holy Spirit to reveal things to you. Seek, and you will find.

> Deuteronomy 4:29 - But from there you will seek the LORD your God, and you will find Him if you seek Him with all your heart and with all your soul.

## March 11

Have you caused your own captivity? In the scripture below, it is talking about being drunk. The people have spent their time with neighbors drinking to excess.

Today, there is much more available. People are in captivity to alcohol, excess sugar, drugs, marijuana, actually this list could be much longer. It also says that people go into captivity from a lack of knowledge.

What is the lack of knowledge? This is a lack of knowledge of the Bible, of what God expects you to do. Think about this, many diseases are caused by your own behavior.

God wants you healthy. Many diseases become a captivity. With the problems mentioned above, the cause of the sickness is your own fault. In these cases, you need to repent. Repent is not just confessing a sin, it means making a change.

God will help you. If you are addicted, God will help you get free. You have to be willing. Some people get instantly delivered. Your knowledge and your will both play a strong role is some healings.

> Isaiah 5:13 - Therefore my people have gone into captivity, because they have no knowledge; their honorable men are famished, and their multitude dried up with thirst.

## March 12

Let Jesus be your example. Jesus always referred back to the Word. He used the Word when He took authority. He used the Word when He ministered to people. He used the Word when He prayed for people to be healed.

You have been given authority over sickness and disease. Many of you have learned that Jesus paid the price for your sickness and disease. This is so true. However, you have an enemy who has rights in darkness. Where you don't know the Word, where you have a lack of knowledge of the Word, the enemy rules.

Are you new to the Word? Don't expect to learn everything in one day. Start with basic teachings, learn scriptures about your authority, and that Jesus paid the price. Learn more!

If you listen to the faith teachers, you will hear all of them tell you that you need to learn the Word, you need to study the Word, you need to use the Word.

You are never too old to learn something new. Learning what the Bible says is more than a lifetime project. You will learn more in heaven!

Hebrews 5:12 - For though by this time you ought to be teachers, you need someone to teach you again the first principles of the oracles of God; and you have come to need milk and not solid food.

## March 13

The world is full of diseases, things that have never been heard of before. There are medications, most of which have side effects. Some of these side effects are new diseases never heard of before.

Many people are always looking for, and trying, the latest cure. Sometimes they are happy with the results, sometimes they are not. Other people want older reliable medications, and there are people who want no medication.

No matter what route you take, and sometimes you may do one thing, other times you may do the other—no matter what you do, seek God, pray, and apply your faith. If you don't use medication, use your faith. If you do take medication, use your faith.

God wants you healed. Sometimes He will tell you to go to the doctor. Sometimes He will say nothing. No matter what, remember, God made the heavens and the earth, He loves you, He wants you well, and nothing is too hard for Him.

Jeremiah 32:17 - Ah, Lord GOD! Behold, You have made the heavens and the earth by Your great power and outstretched arm. There is nothing too hard for You.

By Patricia L. Whipp

## March 14

Can anyone be healed? The answer to that may be no. God wants everyone healed. Some people place themselves in a position that they cannot be. That was their choice.

One reason is unforgiveness. If you refuse to forgive someone, you place yourself in a position that your prayers, including healing, will be hindered.

In the scripture below, the word "eye" is translated elsewhere as conscience. If you are doing something you know is wrong, and you refuse to quit or to do what is right, you have removed yourself from the right to be healed.

Does everyone sin, certainly. Are you one who repents when you realize what you did? Then don't concern yourself about it. Are you one who says, "I don't care, I want to do that," then this says your body may be full of darkness. You give place to sickness.

Some things are not wise, but they are not a sin. You need to seek God and learn what He says. Keep your eye shining. Be a light to others. Receive your healing.

> Luke 11:34 - The lamp of the body is the eye. Therefore, when your eye is good, your whole body also is full of light. But when your eye is bad, your body also is full of darkness.

## March 15

Abraham is an excellent example of what God will do for you. In fact, this example is a healing example! Sarah was barren. God had promised Abraham a son. The son was to be through Sarah. Abraham never gave up. He fully believed. He was going to have a son.

Did Abraham make a mistake? Yes, he had Ishmael. But still he never gave up. When God said that it was to be through Sarah, Abraham never gave up. He had received his son, he didn't know when, but he never gave up.

When you pray, or when others pray for a healing for you, do not give up. If you are fully convinced, and have received it, do not give up. See yourself healed. Talk your healing. Just as Abraham said, "We will be back," as he and Isaac headed up the mountain. You must see and talk yourself healed.

This is the reason many people are not healed. They give up. They do not see it, they do not receive it.

> Romans 4:21 - and being fully convinced that what He had promised He was also able to perform.

## March 16

When you receive a healing, and it is fully manifested, you are often not through. Do not let that be discouraging. You are victorious. You are in charge. You just have to know that, and you may need to take some steps.

After you are fully healed, and resting in your healing, you may receive some symptoms of the same thing again! Don't be discouraged, don't give into those symptoms. The devil is simply trying to see if he can get you trapped again.

You know you are the victor. Stand your ground. He must flee. What if the doctor had told you it might come back? Don't yield to those symptoms. Tell the devil to flee. Use some scriptures as you tell him this. They are like a sword that cuts him.

This is why it is so important to quote healing scriptures out loud to yourself, even when you are well. You are keeping your spirit and your soul built up. They are like a flu shot. They are your booster shot. You must stand firm, the devil must flee.

> James 4:7 - Therefore submit to God. Resist the devil and he will flee from you.

## March 17

Praise God for what He has given us. God has designed healing, He wants you to live a good lifestyle, and to know good health. At times, everyone finds themselves fighting the good fight of faith and getting healed. But that was not God's plan.

We were created in God's image. Our bodies were designed to renew cells throughout the body at night as we sleep. People who do not sleep enough rob themselves of this cell renewal.

If you are living a very healthy life right now, praise God. If you are believing for good health, praise God. Your praise life should be consistent regardless of your physical condition.

God loves you, He provides for you, that includes health. Learn to be consistent in your time with God. Thank Him for what He does for you. Praise Him for what He does for you. Let God be exalted.

> Psalm 18:46 - The LORD lives! Blessed be my Rock! Let the God of my salvation be exalted.

# March 18

When you were born again, did you have to do anything? Yes, you had to hear about Jesus, you had to choose to receive Jesus, you had to accept Him. If you didn't have to do anything, then everyone would be born again, because that is what God wants.

Do you have to do anything to be healed? You have to hear the Word. You have to know that God wants you healed, you have to accept it. With both being born again and with healing, things often go fast. You were not aware of these.

God does not automatically heal you. If He did, no one would be sick, ever. That is what He would like, but look around you, it doesn't happen. As you grow, you are more responsible.

Don't ever forget that Jesus bore your sickness before the cross, just as He bore your sins by going to the cross and fighting for you in hell. He paid the price, He bore your sicknesses and your sins.

So, if you have a sickness try to come on you, make the decision to be healed. Go to the throne, pray, or have people pray for you, take authority over this, and boldly say, the Lord is my helper, my healer, I will not fear—what can be done to me?

Hebrews 13:6 - So we may boldly say: "The LORD is my helper; I will not fear. What can be done to me?"

## March 19

What is truth? God's Word is truth. If you are seeking a healing for yourself or someone else, it is recommended that you find scriptures that you want to stand on. Those are scriptures that can be used for meditation. Those scriptures are medicine.

Once you have scriptures ready, you are ready to pray. Use the scriptures that you have prepared for meditation. Those also are great to use for prayer. Your scriptures should include at least two areas.

One area you want to include is that God heals! God wants you healed. There are many scriptures in the Bible which show this. There are scriptures in both the Old and the New Testaments about God healing.

Another thing you are doing is renewing your mind. So, you want to find scriptures which show what you should look like when you are healed. For example, for a leg problem, scriptures about walking, leaping and running.

Now you are ready, with truth, to call upon God, and to meditate His Word as medicine.

> Psalm 145:18 - The LORD is near to all who call upon Him, to all who call upon Him in truth.

By Patricia L. Whipp

## March 20

How would you like to have a tree of life? That word life does not just mean that you aren't dead, it includes lively, revived, it is a good thing. A wholesome tongue is a tree of life.

Talk life. Talk good things. Talk about good health. Talk that you are healed. You will find that the statement, "You can have what you say," has more truth to it than you realized.

If you talk death, talk bad things, talk sickness and disease, talk about bad things all of the time, find something wrong with every thing, that does damage to your spirit. Learn to control your tongue.

Do you know someone who always finds something wrong with everything? They talk negative all of the time. They are always down. Their health is probably not good.

Learn to speak the good. If you can't think of anything good to say, keep your mouth shut. Say nothing.

God is good. Learn to share the goodness of God with others.

Proverbs 15:4 - A wholesome tongue
is a tree of life, but perverseness in
it breaks the spirit.

## March 21

Are you in need of healing? God wants you healed. He has provided healing for you. Jesus was beaten and died on a cross to pay the price for all healing. With every stripe of the whip He paid the price for healing.

Healing was available to the Jews in the Old Testament. Jesus operated under the Old Testament when He walked the earth. He taught many things, but He always healed people, prayed for people to be well.

There is a far better covenant today, healing is definitely available. We are told in Psalms that God's Word is settled. That includes today.

If you want healing, start with the Bible. Choose healing scriptures. There are many methods. You can pray, believe and trust God. You can have others pray for you. That can be in a church service or on a street corner with a stranger who offers to pray for you.

You can use your authority and take your healing that way. Demand the enemy away from you with that sickness.

No matter how, where, or when, healing is available. Believe and receive your healing. Walk free from sickness and disease.

Psalm 119:89 - Forever, O LORD, Your word is settled in heaven.

## March 22

Do you want healing? It is available. The Bible never changes. People keep coming up with new names, new diseases, but there is nothing that God cannot heal. There is no disease that God cannot undo.

The first thing is, don't be afraid of any disease. It is not bigger than God. Do not even listen to the news media, they probably don't know the Bible. Most likely they do not know your God.

Learn to pray for the news media, and turn the TV off, or to a channel where you can learn something good. God made the heavens and the earth. Do you think man can mess it up so bad that God can't undo it?

Learn to trust God. He loves you with an everlasting love. He wants you healed. He wants you free from all sickness and disease.

Spend time in praise and worship. Thank God for your healing, thank Him for all that He does for you. Thank Him for His love. Tell God that you love Him.

> Psalm 121:2 - My help comes from the LORD, Who made heaven and earth.

## March 23

Healing is from God. God wants you well. When He took the people out of Egypt, He healed everyone before they left. God is so good. He is full of compassion for His people, He is a merciful God.

Have you ever heard anyone say, "God is going to get you for that?" They are not speaking about the God who created heaven and earth. They are talking about a false God. There is so much going on in the world, so many lies. Satan is the liar, and the father of lies.

God wants nothing but the best for you. He wants you walking in peace, enjoying life. Now, He does expect some things from you. He expects you to put Him first. He expects you walking in love towards others. He expects you walking in forgiveness.

Do you know people who consider this unreasonable? I do, but that is just because of their ignorance. Pray for their eyes to be opened.

Praise God and receive your healing.

Psalm 145:8 - The LORD is gracious and full of compassion, slow to anger and great in mercy.

## March 24

Jesus was beaten, He suffered every disease, every sickness you could have for your healing. He went to hell for you, and stripped Satan of all rights to anything for you. The price for your healings has been paid.

Don't ever forget this. You have been given authority over the devil. He can bring sickness to you. He functions in darkness, and where you don't know that you have authority over him, he brings sickness.

Your light is in the Bible. Where you have knowledge of the scriptures, you rule. By knowing that Jesus suffered for you, you have knowledge. Isaiah 53:4-5. That alone gives you light.

Do not cast away your confidence. Hold tight to the knowledge that you have authority over any disease or sickness that may come your way. Hold on to that knowledge, and take authority over any problems that plague you.

> Hebrews 10:35 - Therefore do not cast away your confidence, which has great reward.

## March 25

As you take your healing, regardless of the steps used, sometimes it seems like things are not going right. Many times, it is easy to step into doubt! Cast that aside. God does not expect you to be perfect, and He does want you well.

Learn to rest in God. Continue reading your Bible, continue meditating on the scriptures you are standing on. Those things are food for your spirit and they keep your faith built up.

But rest. Know you have done what you need to do, know that God is faithful. Know that Jesus paid the price for your healing as He went to the cross.

When you prayed, when you took authority, you cried out to God. You have done your part. Know that God performs all things for you.

> Psalm 57:2 - I will cry out to God Most High, to God who performs all things for me

## March 26

It was prophesied by Isaiah what Jesus would do. The fact that He took our infirmities and bore our sicknesses, that was prophesied centuries before it became a fact. For centuries people knew it was to happen. It is now a fact. We know it happened.

This is proof that God wants you healed. This is how you know that all sickness and disease have been paid for. This gives you the confidence that you have every right to demand that Satan take all sickness and disease from your body.

This is more light for you to walk in. Satan can not reign where you have light. He has no power in light. He only rules in darkness. When you have no knowledge, he can bring problems to you.

Once you have the light of the Word, you can take authority over the devil, and he MUST flee. He has no power in light. Take your authority, demand your health, and walk in your health.

> Matthew 8:17 - that it might be fulfilled which was spoken by Isaiah the prophet, saying: "He Himself took our infirmities and bore our sicknesses."

## March 27

Stand on the Word of God. What does that mean? It means that when you pick a scripture that you are going to use for prayer, you don't move. You acquire patience, you believe and don't quit.

Psalm 91 is a great psalm to use. It includes health. This tells you that no evil, no plague, or sickness, shall come near your home. Once you have prayed, you hold fast to your prayer. Don't doubt, or waver. Don't give up.

God cannot lie. He has promised that no evil shall befall you, nor any plague come near your dwelling. Your head has to be renewed, your spirit fed. Your faith built up.

This is why you don't wait till the evil comes, you start when things are good. It is easier to maintain good, than to start to fight after the evil has come.

> Psalm 91:10 - No evil shall befall you, nor shall any plague come near your dwelling;

By Patricia L. Whipp

# March 28

Why isn't the manifestation of healing always instant? How much longer? I can't go on! We hear these statements often. When you are doing what God has told you to do, when your faith is set, you need to hold tight. One minister has said, when you are ready to wait as long as necessary, it will come quickly.

I cannot give you a full explanation, but I fully believe that the answer to your prayer is sent to you when you pray. God wants you well. We know that the angel was on the way to Daniel the day Daniel prayed. But it took time for the angel to get there.

One of the first people to ask for prayer in one community was miraculously healed, but had to deal with bad feelings about the length of time it took. We see miracle healing meetings where some things happen instantly, and some healings start that day.

Some of the miracles started years before. The person has been meditating healing scriptures for a long time and had prayed previously.

What I do know, God wants you healed. The healing was sent with the first prayer. You must trust God, you must be steadfast, sing and give praise for the answer.

> Psalm 57:7 - My heart is steadfast,
> O God, my heart is steadfast; I will
> sing and give praise.

# March 29

Are you weary, are you tired? If that is your normal condition, that alone can make you sick. God did not plan for you to toil, or be exhausted all the time. There may be seasons where it is necessary to miss rest and sleep, but not on a regular basis.

God has a rest for you. If you are believing for something, and this includes a healing, you pray, and you rest. Let God do the work for you. You can't mend a broken bone, you can't heal cancer.

Confessing scriptures is not toil, it is not work. Scriptures are medicine. So when you are confessing scriptures, consider it taking medicine. It should be refreshing to you.

There are times when I have been busy doing work, and reading the scriptures out loud totally energizes me. The Israelites did not hear that. They did not understand, so they did not hear what God was telling them.

Learn to walk in divine healing. Learn to walk the way God tells you to walk, and enjoy the rest that God has for you.

> Isaiah 28:12 - To whom He said, "This is the rest with which You may cause the weary to rest," and, "This is the refreshing"; yet they would not hear.

## March 30

God has given you life. Life is living healthy, living well. Sickness is not a part of the life that God gives to you. Sickness can lead to death, it often does not allow you to do the things God has for you.

What leads to life is the fear of the Lord. That word fear is not the word for scared. It is a reverence; an awe of the Lord; a recognition of what God has done for you; a total respect for the life God has placed in you.

When you have this life, you will live in a satisfaction, a peace, a pleasant life. You will not be constantly looking for something else. You will be at rest with your life.

This also says that you will not be visited with evil. That does not mean that you will be totally left alone by the enemy, but it means that evil cannot be put upon you. You have power over all power of the enemy.

So, to have a healthy life, to enjoy your life, have a reverence of God. Keep God first place in your life. Those are all things which will help you to maintain a good life. Spend time praising God. Spend time thanking Him for what He has done for you.

> Proverbs 19:23 - The fear of the LORD leads to life, and he who has it will abide in satisfaction; he will not be visited with evil.

## March 31

Joshua, as his time was coming to an end, spoke to the people. He spent time giving them instructions concerning how they were to continue living. He said, "… As for me and my house, we will serve the Lord." (Joshua 24:15)

The people answered that they would continue to serve the Lord. We may be under a different covenant, we have grace being strongly taught, we have a promise of healing because of what Jesus suffered for us before the crucifixion.

That is not changed—we need to make this commitment, "As for me and my house, I will serve the Lord." Healing is not automatic. It is definitely available, it is promised, but if you are serving other gods, what do you think?

No, you will not be perfect. You will make mistakes. There are times when you will sin. Check yourself, is your goal to serve God? Do you repent when you realize you goofed? That is all God is asking of you. Not perfection, but willingness is needed.

> Joshua 24:16 - So the people answered and said: "Far be it from us that we should forsake the LORD to serve other gods;

## April 1

Abraham's blessings are in Deuteronomy chapter 28. The first 14 verses are the blessings, the rest of the chapter, verses 15-68, are the curses. Sometimes, it is easier to say what a blessing is by listing the curses.

ALL sickness and disease are under the curses. Therefore, good health is under the blessings. As a Christian, even if you are a Gentile, you walk under the blessings of Abraham.

When you know the truth, it will set you free. The truth is that you have all rights to good health! God wants you healthy. That is His desire. A point that many people miss is that you have to receive your healing.

Non-Christians and baby Christians get healing dumped on them. Praise God. But as you grow up, you need to learn to apply your faith. You cannot please God without faith. You have to receive. It's there, waiting for you. Receive your healing.

> Galatians 3:14 - that the blessing of Abraham might come upon the Gentiles in Christ Jesus, that we might receive the promise of the Spirit through faith.

## April 2

In the scripture below it says, "The Lord was ready to save me…." In some versions of the Bible, the word used that was translated 'save' is translated 'heal.' Normally, any time the word 'save' is used referring to humans, it can also be translated heal.

This says therefore we will sing…. That is excellent. Learn to praise God for healing you. Learn to thank Him for healing. God wants you well. He wants you healed. After this was written, God sent Jesus to earth for you.

When are you healed? When it manifests? No. You are healed when it is prayed for, and you have received it. The manifestation may be later, but the healing takes place when it is received.

This is something that needs to be understood. Praise God for your healing. Sing to God for your healing. Thank God for your healing.

> Isaiah 38:20 - "The LORD was ready to save me; therefore we will sing my songs with stringed instruments all the days of our life, in the house of the LORD."

## April 3

Praise God! We serve a God who loves us very much. He wants nothing but the best for us. He wants us healthy, totally healed. That statement is true from birth, to 120 years old. God supplies good health.

I had heard that people say this, but someone asked me about a year ago, "How will we die if we don't get sick?" You just give up the spirit.

The choice is yours, the ability to let go is yours. The one question you need to ask is, "Have I accomplished what God wants me to do yet? Am I finished?"

Paul shows us that. He had been through a lot (2 Corinthians 11:23-28), but he knew that he had more work to do. People still needed him to teach them about what God wants, what He expects of us.

In the scripture below, if you are sick, petition God, pray for your healing. Then accept it. Know you have the answer. There are many scriptures that tell us, God never fails.

Learn to trust God, and let the healing manifest in your life.

> 1 John 5:15 - And if we know that He hears us, whatever we ask, we know that we have the petitions that we have asked of Him.

## April 4

Have you been listening to the prophets lately? They are saying that healing miracles are here now. Miracles like there have never been seen anywhere. They are here. Have you heard the reports? Healing miracles are here.

There is a minister in Africa whose elbow had been shot. An artificial elbow was put in. It was very painful. God told him one night He was going to do something special for him. The next morning he woke up, and he had a new elbow in his arm. The artificial elbow was on the bed right beside him.

A woman with leukemia woke up one morning with blood everywhere, in the bed, on her clothes, on the floor. She had received a transfusion that night. No leukemia in her body.

Miracles are here. We need to pray to keep them going, we need to pray for healings. We also need to pray for salvations. Pray for these things to happen around the world.

Pray for revival. It is happening, but prayers will keep it going. Pray for people to be born again, pray for healings. Pray for these to occur around the world, every country, every nation.

> Amos 3:7 - Surely the Lord GOD does nothing, unless He reveals His secret to His servants the prophets.

## April 5

God told the Israelites several times, and in at least three books, that He has set before them the way of life and the way of death.

You will find the same is true today. You have a way of life, and a way of death. Jesus is the way of life, the world is the way of death.

The way of life includes, and has always included, health. A Greek word often used for life includes every area of life needed for a good life. A good life includes health. The choice has been given to you.

That can be harsh if you let it. You need to renew your mind. You need to adjust your thinking.

Cancer. That is a name. God can, and will, heal it. It doesn't need to take a long time. It can, but that is not God's best.

Learn what the Bible says, and go for God's best. Go for full health. Strive to walk in divine health.

> Jeremiah 21:8 - "Now you shall say to this people, 'Thus says the LORD: "Behold, I set before you the way of life and the way of death.

## April 6

Did you know that God set the age of man to 120 years? That is in Genesis 6. That is the life span you can expect to reach if you desire. The places that say that man was only to live to 80 were speaking about the Israelites as they were going to the promised land. Their age was limited because of their attitude and disobedience.

Does that change some of your thinking? Moses lived to 120, and his eyes were still good. As one version put it, there was still a spring in his step. He was still healthy and vigorous. That was not just because he was Moses. That is what is available to you.

Did your ancestors die by 80, so you think you should also? Do not go by when your ancestors died. Maybe they lived longer, but if not, that does not mean that you can't live to 120. God needs you here!

God wants you well. He needs people who will witness, who will tell others about Jesus, and who will pray in these end days. Are you willing to commit to this? Set your faith, take your stand, and continue in God's army.

> Deuteronomy 34:7 - Moses was one hundred and twenty years old when he died. His eyes were not dim nor his natural vigor diminished.

## April 7

Christians are grafted into the seed of Abraham. The blessings are all available to them. Included in the blessings are all healing.

Jesus paid the price for you when He went to the cross. Also, you have blessings promised to you when you use your faith.

Faith is something God likes. In fact, it is impossible to please God without faith. (Hebrews 11:6 ) He wants you to use your faith here on earth. I have heard it said that faith is the currency used in heaven.

Learn to apply your faith for healing. As you grow, God expects more of you. He expects you to apply your faith. You can start by applying your faith when others pray for your healing.

There is an all out war going on in the heavenlies. Satan may try to bring several different illnesses to you. Just take authority, and demand your rights. Watch each problem the enemy brings fail. Sometimes he is a slow learner, but you are the victor.

Praise God for your healing, apply your faith and watch your healing be fully completed.

> Galatians 3:9 - So then those who are of faith are blessed with believing Abraham.

## April 8

It would be very easy to misunderstand the use of the scripture below; judgment in the house of God. Is God going to judge you? Is God going to make you sick? Positively not. Then who, or how, are you going to be judged?

You actually bring problems on yourself. That is what Job did. When Job realized what he had done wrong, and followed God's instructions, he was healed, and everything was restored to him.

Think about it, if you drink too much alcohol, you will be drunk. If you eat too much food, you will be sick. Many times you bring things on yourself. The same can be true of your health. God wants you well. He wants you healed. But when you ignore His warnings, you can make yourself sick.

The same is true in many areas, if you watch scary movies, you can be afraid. God did not give you fear, that is the devil's territory.

God says that His people are destroyed by a lack of knowledge; a lack of knowledge of what? Knowledge of what the Bible says. The Bible is truth and light. God is light. Use light to destroy sickness, to destroy all power of evil.

> 1 Peter 4:17 - For the time has come for judgment to begin at the house of God; and if it begins with us first, what will be the end of those who do not obey the gospel of God?

## April 9

God wants you well. We know He gave us His Word, that we might be healed. He did that so, in part, people might be delivered from the destructions that they put themselves into. God wants them delivered from doing harmful things to their body.

This can be many things. This can be wrong eating, bad habits, for example, smoking. There is no form of smoking that is good for you. Tobacco, marijuana, both are bad for your health. Articles are now appearing on the internet about how good marijuana is for you. Don't be ensnared with what you read.

Spending time praising God, spending time in true worship, these are ways to spend your time that are beneficial to your body as well as to your soul and spirit. This will give an opportunity for healing.

Always keep first in your thoughts, God crowns you with lovingkindness and tender mercies. He wants you healthy. He gave His Son for your salvation, and for your health, as well as for your life on this earth.

> Psalm 103:4 - Who redeems your life from destruction, Who crowns you with lovingkindness and tender mercies,

## April 10

Are you at peace? If you are not at peace, you are probably stressed, upset, overly busy. Those will all lead to sickness. Heart problems, stroke, high blood pressure and other sicknesses can be related to not being at peace.

God tells you to seek first the Kingdom of God. Are you seeking that first? If you are not, that is where you need to start. You can be sure that is true because that is what God tells you is first!

If you are walking in the Kingdom of God, you have righteousness. Jesus has made unto you His righteousness. You can know from Isaiah that you will then have peace, quietness and assurance.

Seems like that gives you a pattern to follow. Do you have a stressful job? One which you are constantly busy and get no rest? Seek God. You could look for another job, but God can direct your steps and show you how to be at peace in stressful situations.

In everything, keep the plan to seek the Kingdom of God first, then enjoy the benefits you will receive from the Kingdom of God.

> Isaiah 32:17 - The work of righteousness will be peace, and the effect of righteousness, quietness and assurance forever.

## April 11

The words of your mouth are very important. Many people do not realize this. They cause their own disasters, including sickness. They see something on TV and speak worry over it. They hear about a disease going around and talk about it.

Words are the start of everything. Words were the start of the big bang which scientists now know started the universe. God said, "Light be," and there was light. It started and is still going.

In the Kingdom, when Jesus reigns, people will know to not say, "I am sick." They will know if something is not right, all they have to do is speak to it. They will know how to speak things into being.

Learn to control your words and your thoughts. As you do this, you will find your life is much better! Speaking right words makes a big difference. This helps stop any sickness, and helps you to walk in divine health.

> Isaiah 33:24 - And the inhabitant will not say, "I am sick"; the people who dwell in it will be forgiven their iniquity.

## April 12

Do you have a problem with hearing, or with seeing? God wants both healed. This scripture may be referring to the spirit. Seeing in the spirit, and hearing in the spirit, but God is also interested in the physical as well as the spiritual.

Learn to observe what is going on around you. God wants you healed. There are so many scriptures which state that. God has paid a very high price for the health of a Christian. He has always wanted His people well. He healed the Israelites when they left Egypt.

There is healing in the scriptures. Learn to use the Bible, use scriptures. Use scriptures that say God will heal. Use scriptures that God wants you healed. Also use scriptures that paint a picture of you healed.

The scripture used here is one that paints a picture of you healed. What do you do with these scriptures? Read them out loud. Seeing them is important. Hearing them is important.

Hearing scriptures builds faith. Seeing scriptures is actually healing to you. The scriptures are medicine to your flesh.

> Isaiah 35:5 - Then the eyes of the blind shall be opened, and the ears of the deaf shall be unstopped.

## April 13

Are you praying for healing? God wants His people healed. He provides healing for everyone, but He wants His people healed. What do you have to do? For one thing, you have to believe that He wants you healed.

Keeping yourself single-minded is vital to your healing. What does single-minded mean? It means you can't doubt. You can't think that He might want you sick a little longer to teach you something. You can't wonder if you caused God to be doing this. God is love, God is kind, gentle, and wants the best for you.

Maintaining a reverence for God, keeping God first place in your heart and mind, is very important. Praise and worship of the Most High is something that helps you to do this. If you can't, question yourself. Do you need to forgive God for something?

God is not upset if you are angry with Him, but you hurt yourself anytime you are in unforgiveness. No matter who you are not forgiving—someone else, yourself, or God, you must forgive.

Praise God, thank Him for His love, and receive what He has for you.

> Psalm 34:9 - Oh, fear the LORD, you His saints! There is no want to those who fear Him.

## April 14

When you are receiving a healing, you usually need to be peaceful, resting, and slowed down. Your body has to work as it is healing. It doesn't need you being active and using all of your energy.

Learn to rest, to be peaceful, and to give your body a chance to do its work. Give it a chance to build up your strength. Your strength is something that often goes when there is sickness going on in your body.

Learn to be quiet and confident. Know that Jesus has paid the price for your healing. Know that healing is there and at work in your body. Have complete confidence in the work which is being done.

As you do this, your strength will return. Have you ever heard people say, "I am catching a cold."? I have asked people why they are catching it! Why didn't they let it go right by them? Don't ever let the words, "I am catching…any disease," come out of your mouth.

Learn to say, "I am healed." As you receive your healing, in complete confidence that it is there, your strength will return.

> Isaiah 30:15 - For thus says the Lord GOD, the Holy One of Israel: "In returning and rest you shall be saved; in quietness and confidence shall be your strength."…

## April 15

Was Jesus ever sick when He was on earth? No! Do you think that God the Father, or Jesus, are ever sick in heaven? No! There is no sickness in heaven. Sickness is something which the devil brought to man on earth.

When you walk with God, you are justified by His grace. Justified, what does that mean? From looking at the Greek word used, it appears that you are made righteous by His grace. If you are made righteous, then sickness has no right being on you!

Whenever sickness tries to come on you, take authority! It has to leave. Don't blame yourself if it takes time to get it off of you. Don't get under condemnation if there is sickness in your body. Don't take on more junk that does not belong to you.

You are in a war. Your enemy does not fight fair, he does not use rules, but he does have to flee. Stand your ground. Know that you are the winner, that the victory is yours. Rest in the knowledge that you are the victor.

> Romans 3:24 - being justified freely by His grace through the redemption that is in Christ Jesus,

## April 16

God has made many promises to you. What some people do not realize is that the devil steals the Word, he steals those promises from you. You have to find the promises and claim them. You have to stand firm on them.

One of the promises is healing. That is so strong. There are so many places, both in the Old and the New Testaments, where you can find scriptures telling you that healing is yours. The prophesy that Jesus would die on the cross in Isaiah shows you that He gave His body for your health.

Once again, you have to claim it. The psalm below is a promise that God will heal you if you pray. It is best if you use scriptures when you pray. No matter what you are praying for, remind God from His Word what it says. Doing that acts as a sword on the devil.

You are in a war. There is no question of that. It was not your choice, you were born at a time in history when the war is going on. The war started the day that Adam ate the apple. It will continue until after the seven years of tribulation.

Read the back of the book. Know that you are a winner.

Psalm 66:19 - But certainly God has heard me; He has attended to the voice of my prayer.

## April 17

God wants you healed. He has always wanted His people healed, but for the Christians He has done even more than was available for people under the Old Testament. God is light. Knowledge of the Word of God gives you light of the Word.

God has sent His first-begotten Son, Jesus, to earth for you. Jesus functioned under Old Testament rules, but He healed everyone who came to Him and wanted healing. He did not turn down anyone. He did not tell anyone to stay sick longer.

All of this should make it clear to you that healing is available. God wants you healed. You may need to learn a little bit of what the Word says. You may need to apply your faith. However, God has given you faith.

What must you do? Praise God. Thank Him for your healing. Do you do this before it manifests? Yes. Once you have been prayed for, or you have prayed, start thanking God. Praise Him. Worship Him. Do these before, and after, the manifestation of the healing.

> Colossians 1:12 - giving thanks to the Father who has qualified us to be partakers of the inheritance of the saints in the light.

## April 18

Cancer? Is that a word to be afraid of? The only thing that can hurt you is if you die without receiving Jesus. If you received Jesus, you have been given a measure of faith. What you need to do is start using your faith, exercise it. Help it to grow.

There is no disease that cannot be cured. There is nothing too difficult for God to heal. There is no deformity that God cannot straighten, there are no missing parts that God cannot replace.

I have been told that there is a warehouse in heaven of spare parts. Use your faith. Faith does not quit. Faith does not give up. If you were believing for something besides healing, I would say you need to find supporting scriptures.

There are supporting scriptures for healing. Most of these have been included in this book. Pain must bow it's knee to the name of Jesus. Jesus suffered all sickness and all pain for you.

As you are exercising your faith, spend time praising God and thanking Him for your healing.

> Luke 17:6 - So the Lord said, "If you have faith as a mustard seed, you can say to this mulberry tree, 'Be pulled up by the roots and be planted in the sea,' and it would obey you.

By Patricia L. Whipp

## April 19

Your flesh, your heart, they can fail. They can have problems, but God is your strength, and yours forever. If you are sick, God is always there. He wants you well. He wants you strong. He wants you healed.

Don't claim a sickness. There is nothing God cannot do for you. Draw from God. Draw from His strength. He is the strength of your heart. Draw from that. Stand your ground from the enemy who is trying to make you sick.

Satan's time is running out, and he is doing all he can to stop his end. A part of that is trying to make God's children sick. If you don't believe in Satan, you had better. He is your enemy, and you have authority over him.

Keep God as your source at all times. Keep your eyes and ears on Him. Do not believe other reports. Doctors do the best they know how. If they are a Christian, drawing from God, praise God for them. If their report is negative, know that God has a better report.

Praise God for your healing, go forth as the redeemed in praise and thanksgiving.

> Ephesians 3:16 - that He would grant you, according to the riches of His glory, to be strengthened with might through His Spirit in the inner man,

# April 20

Are you believing for a healing? Have you been prayed for, either you prayed, or others prayed and are in agreement? Have you received your healing? That is easy. After prayer, you say, "I receive." Then it is yours.

You are a conqueror. That means in everything. There is nothing that the enemy can bring against you that Jesus has not already conquered. You share in what Jesus has conquered. Therefore you are more than a conqueror.

That includes health. There is no disease, infirmity, sickness of any kind for which the price has not been paid. Therefore it is yours. You are more than a conqueror. The price has been paid.

When you get a hold of this, when you realize this truth, you should be shouting. Shout for joy. You are more than a conqueror. Praise God! The victory is won, the price has been paid. Healing is yours.

> Romans 8:37 - Yet in all these things we are more than conquerors through Him who loved us.

## April 21

Are you believing for a healing for yourself or other people? That covers almost everybody. A family member, a co-worker, a neighbor, a friend, you may be praying for some of these people.

As you pray, think about all that God does for you. Everyone of these words in the scripture below can lead to health or healing. God wants you healed, He is the one who formed you, He is the one who wants you well.

This verse gives you much to hold onto. If you are praying for yourself, or anyone else, what more could you want? If you are praying for someone else, you might want to share this verse with them.

Rock, fortress, those will protect you, be it a sickness, or a storm, these will hold you. They will protect you from the elements and from all that is raging around you. Your deliverer, your strength, God will deliver you from any sickness, and will strengthen you.

God is your shield, and He designed your salvation. Praise God. Thank Him, spend time worshiping Him, praise Him.

> Psalm 18:2 - The LORD is my rock and my fortress and my deliverer; my God, my strength, in whom I will trust; my shield and the horn of my salvation, my stronghold.

## April 22

Praise God for His promises to you, for His healing power, for watching over you in the day and in the night. God truly loves you and protects you. Psalm 91 is a wonderful psalm for you to use on a daily basis. It is great on good days and on bad days.

If you let God protect you, man cannot hurt you. You do have to take steps. First, you should have accepted Jesus as your Lord and Savior. Then, you have to keep the Bible as your source. The scriptures are medicine for you.

If you go the world's way, then you should fear. Man, through the help of God's enemy, can do a lot to you if you ignore God. You can be hurt, sick, down and out. Don't go the world's way! Stick with God.

God loves you. Love God. Keep Him first in your life. He told you to seek first the Kingdom. Do that.

The Word says to be absent from the body is to be present with God. (2 Corinthians 5:8) So, even if something did happen to you, you will end up in a better place. When you get that fully built into your spirit, then you know nothing can hurt you.

> Psalm 118:6 - The LORD is on my side; I will not fear. What can man do to me?

113

# April 23

God loves you. He loves you with an everlasting love. God loves you as much as He loves Jesus. That is hard to believe, but that is what the Bible says, so it must be true. Learn to love God, to trust God, to believe He loves you.

God wants you well. He does not ever make you sick; He does not delay healing to teach you anything. The reason you often learn things while you are sick is because it forces you to slow down. At that time, you turn to God.

When you are born again, you have overcome the world. You have the victory over the world, that includes victory over all sickness. Why do you have this victory? Because God has given you faith. Start exercising your faith. Learn to trust God.

Hold tight to the knowledge that God wants you well. Hold tight to the knowledge that healing is yours. It is available for you.

Find scriptures that help you to see this truth. Read scriptures out loud every day. Scriptures are medicine for you.

> 1 John 5:4 - For whatever is born of God overcomes the world. And this is the victory that has overcome the world—our faith.

## April 24

When Adam was created, he was designed to last forever. His body regenerated itself, cells died and were replaced with new cells. Our bodies have a measure of this. As you sleep, your body does renew a lot of cells. For people who cut their sleep short, their body wears out faster.

However, when Adam fell, when he turned the lease to the earth over to Satan, many things changed. Our bodies tend to not work as well as they should. Satan has corrupted many things which has caused diseases to attack us.

As a result, your flesh at times will fail. Your heart can wear out. The Good News is that God has always wanted His people well, He heals people. Jesus bore your sickness and disease when He was beaten before He went to the cross.

Keep God first in your life. Seek first the Kingdom of God. God is the strength of your heart, God will keep your heart strong. Keep God as your portion forever.

Psalm 73:26 - My flesh and my heart fail; but God is the strength of my heart and my portion forever.

## April 25

Do you have problems breathing? God caused dry bones to come together, He put skin on the bones, and He caused breath to enter the dry bones. This was shown to Ezekiel. What a picture for you. Meditate on this scripture.

When you are seeking healing, you use scriptures that God heals. God wants you healed. It is also good to have a scripture that paints a picture of you completely healed, and the desired results of your prayers manifested. That is true for any area, not just health.

The scripture below paints a beautiful picture for someone with breathing problems. God will cause breath to enter you, and you shall live. What a beautiful picture to see as you are meditating on scriptures.

The use of scriptures is so important for every day life. Scriptures are your life source. God gave you pictures throughout the Bible. Learn to find them, and stand on these scriptures.

> Ezekiel 37:5 - Thus says the Lord GOD to these bones: "Surely I will cause breath to enter into you, and you shall live.

## April 26

Have you been healed? Then say so. Scriptures say, "Let the redeemed say so." (Psalm 107:2) If you are healed, let the healed say so. Have you been prayed for, for healing? How do you receive your healing? You say, "I receive." That simple.

So, unless you deny it, your healing is on it's way. It does not have to manifest immediately. It is on it's way. As an example, let's say you have a broken bone. If you go to the doctor, it will take weeks to heal.

Often, God speeds up the healing, not necessarily; but it is on it's way. The process is started. The time involved is not really important. What is important is your words, your actions. You need to see yourself healed.

If someone tells you they are going to buy a you a new suit, do you thank them when you receive it, or when they say they are buying it? You had better thank them when they say they are buying it.

Learn to do the same with God. Meditate on His work. Thank Him for your healing. Talk about the things God has done, and the things God is doing. Praise God for your healing.

Psalm 77:12 - I will also meditate on all Your work, and talk of Your deeds.

## April 27

If you haven't heard of these people, they are from the Bible. There was a woman with an issue of blood. She had heard of Jesus. She had spent all of her money on doctors and decided she was going to Jesus and she would be healed. She was.

In the Old Testament, a woman had provided a room for a prophet. She and her husband had no children. The prophet spoke, and they had a child. Then one day the child died. The woman went to the prophet. He came and prayed for the child, and the child rose and lived.

We are children of a great God. There is nothing He won't do for you. He wants you well, healthy, and delighting in Him. Look at your own life. Has God done things for you? If you are born again, He has done a marvelous thing for you. If you are not born again, you need to be.

There is nothing God will not do for you. He has given you authority to move mountains. (Mark 11:23) That means any healing is available for you. Quote the following scripture to God as a praise and a thank you.

> Psalm 86:10 - For You are great, and do wondrous things; You alone are God.

# April 28

Salvation comes from God. Do you have any idea what is included in salvation? Healing is included. God wants His people healed. He wants them healthy, He wants them well. There are many other things included.

There are times when people are healed when they are born again. Not often, but it does happen. Many people receive prayer for healing soon after they are born again. At that time, they haven't learned to doubt God, so they are more likely to be instantly healed.

Learn to trust God, to believe God wants the best for you. Sing to God, shout joyfully to God. Do this in praise and worship of God. Don't loose your faith, your hope. The enemy will lie to you and tell you He doesn't care about you. Since Satan is the father of lies, learn to recognize that as a lie.

Things aren't always instant. In this day of microwaves, instant pudding, and frozen dinners, we are not accustomed to waiting. (Unless you are on hold on the phone!)

Trust God, sing praises to God, shout for joy to the Rock of our salvation. Don't be moved by what you see, only be moved by what God has told you in the Bible.

> Psalm 95:1 - Oh come, let us sing to the LORD! Let us shout joyfully to the Rock of our salvation.

119

## April 29

Meditating scriptures is a very good thing to do. If you are sick, this is medicine to your body, and it is food and nourishment to your spirit. If you are well, this is a road to divine health for the same reasons.

Quoting some healing scriptures daily is good for you. You should quote scriptures in several areas of your life daily. This helps to keep your faith built up in those areas of your life as well.

Then, with a strong spirit, your spirit can sustain you through the healing of your sickness. You have food in your spirit, your mind renewed in the areas you have meditated on, and your faith built in those areas.

If your spirit is not fed, it can be much harder for you to recover when you get sick. Not only that, but others around you are not comfortable with you.

Learn to maintain your spirit, to keep it built up, well fed.

Proverbs 18:14 - The spirit of a man will sustain him in sickness, but who can bear a broken spirit?

## April 30

Do you realize that God wants you healed? From the beginning of the Bible to the end, there are scriptures talking about people being healed.

What will add long life and peace to you? This is from Proverbs, it is talking about God's Word, and following God's instructions. Some translations use the word Law. It is not referring to being legalistic. The Word was called the Law.

Scriptures are medicine to your flesh. Scriptures are healing. Many people do not realize this. Meditating the Word is not being legalistic, it is not being into works. Meditating the Word is being a doer of the Word. God is always pleased when people are doers of His Word.

It is also health to you, and as stated in the scripture below, it will add days to your life and peace. Is your life busy, stressful, in turmoil? Realize that something is wrong. Slow down, figure out what you need to drop, and get back to the basics.

Let God lead you and teach you what He has for you, and what steps He suggests for you.

Proverbs 3:2 - For length of days and long life and peace they will add to you.

By Patricia L. Whipp

## May 1

God is always available to help you. He wants you healed. He wants you free from all things that are unhealthy for you. This includes anxiety, stress, and fear. These are all things that are not from God, but can cause sickness.

Fear is something to really check yourself about. Fear is the opposite of faith. Just as faith is from God, fear is from Satan. The minute you realize you are doing something out of fear, catch yourself, and stop it immediately.

God is your help and your shield. God will direct your steps. If you have committed yourself to God, then trust him to guide you.

At times, He authors the thought in your mind such as, "I need to go to this store now." When you get there, you may find yourself witnessing to someone. You may never realize that it was not your thought, it was God who got you there.

In the same way, God will direct your path to keep you healthy. I wanted to see someone about a problem I was having. The person I would normally have seen was sick. A friend recommended someone else. It turned out he was an expert in the field of a disease I didn't even know I had, but the first test he did clearly showed it. It was greatly reduced in a week. God wants the best for you.

Psalm 33:20 - Our soul waits for the LORD; He is our help and our shield.

## May 2

Have you prayed for a healing? Then know it is yours. Do not be moved by how you feel, by what you see, by what is happening. Only be moved by the Word of God.

Praise God for your healing. Find scriptures that minister to you and read them, as you would take medicine. Scriptures are medicine to you, they bring about healing. Speaking them out loud is the only way to activate them. It is called meditation.

Note that Daniel did the same thing. This was for something other than healing, but the actions are the same. As a custom, Daniel prayed three times a day. Jewish custom said morning, noon, and night.

Doing this on a regular basis, through out the day, is excellent. It keeps the scripture alive in your mind, your spirit, and it keeps you in communion with God on a regular basis through out the day. Do not forget to praise God as well as meditate scriptures.

> Daniel 6:10 - Now when Daniel knew that the writing was signed, he went home. And in his upper room, with his windows open toward Jerusalem, he knelt down on his knees three times that day, and prayed and gave thanks before his God, as was his custom since early days.

## May 3

Are you a believer?  Then Jesus said that you will do greater works than He did when He goes to the Father.  He has gone to the Father.  That was many centuries ago.  So, what greater works should you be doing?

Heal the sick.  That is where many minds go.  There were other things that Jesus did, but let's stay with this point.  You should be laying hands on the sick and watching them recover.  That is not just a pastor's job, or any other of the offices.

Are you afraid they won't get well?  That is not your job.  Your job is to pray for the sick, believe, and know that they will recover.  It does not have to be instantly.  The healing is there, and is working.

Think of a broken bone, it takes time.  God can speed it up, but does not always.  Don't ignore people because of your pride, or your fear. Sometimes, a person is not healed because they don't receive the healing.

Don't let people be robbed because you wouldn't follow the Bible.  Learn to be a doer.

> John 14:12 - "Most assuredly, I say to you, he who believes in Me, the works that I do he will do also; and greater works than these he will do, because I go to My Father.

## May 4

In the scripture below, many translations use the word "thoughts" instead of anxieties. Either word is fine for talking about divine health. To walk in divine health, you cannot have anxieties! If you have negative thoughts a lot, forget divine health.

Fear, panic, being anxious, constantly upset, these all lead to sickness. Ask any doctor, any medical practitioner, and they will all agree, these things lead to sickness of some kind.

Jesus gave you His peace. Learn to walk in peace. Learn to live in peace, practice peace. This may sound weird to you, but you have peace in you. Jesus gave it to you, it is inside you.

I actually call it forth. I used to do it for myself. In praying for others, there are times when I am led to speak to peace in the person I am praying for. I tell the peace to rise.

Let God show you where you are anxious, where you need to get things out of you. Find scriptures that you need to meditate on to have peace rise up in you.

On the freeway, in what looked like a total accident situation, God had me wrapped in a blanket of peace. I saw a space open up and moved over. Let God do that for you.

> Psalm 139:23 - Search me, O God, and know my heart; try me, and know my anxieties;

By Patricia L. Whipp

# May 5

God wants you healed, spirit, soul, and body. There are people who don't study the Bible, or even read God's Word. They may be healthy in their body, but their spirit and soul are blind and deaf. They do not understand the Word. When they hear truth, they don't know what they are hearing.

Understanding of the Word comes from having light on what you see. God's people perish for a lack of light, or understanding, of the Word. (Hosea 4:6) Darkness is where Satan rules. If you don't understand that healing is yours, then you give place to sickness.

Faith comes from hearing. If you don't understand what you hear, then you don't have light on the Word. Sickness in your spirit, soul, and body can come from not hearing, or not understanding, the Word. Then you don't have faith to fight sickness.

Make a decision, decide you will believe the Word. Read the Word. When you see pastors who are successful, they have healing happen in their church, they explain the Word, they don't say, "You never know what God is going to do," or "God is in control." Listen to those pastors.

Adam gave control of the world to Satan 6,000 years ago. The Bible tells you what God has done, He has given authority to the body of Christ to pray, take authority, and get things done.

As you grow, your spirit will alert you when you are hearing teachings to ignore. Grow with God, hear and see what the Bible says.

Isaiah 42:18 - "Hear, you deaf; and look, you blind, that you may see.

## May 6

God wants you healed, He wants you walking in divine health. God loves you. When you wake up to the love that God has for you, you will realize how much God wants you healed. In the verse below, He is promising the covenant He had with David to you.

God tells you so many places in the Bible that He wants you healed. He made promises to many of the Old Covenant rulers. How much more has He given to the New Testament saints? Get this solid in your soul and heart.

Jesus died on the cross, in part for your health, for your life on earth, also, for your salvation, for you to have eternity in heaven. Even in the Old Testament, they were assured of going to heaven. The words "your soul shall live" implies that promise.

Serve God, serve the One who created man, who wants man with Him for eternity.

> Isaiah 55:3 - Incline your ear, and come to Me. Hear, and your soul shall live; and I will make an everlasting covenant with you— the sure mercies of David.

## May 7

Do you thank God for healing when you are praying for a healing? Do you thank God for divine health when there is nothing wrong? You should. The verse below says to give thanks in everything.

When you pray for healing, you know you are praying in confidence because there are so many places where He promises you to be healed. That is God's will, that is God's best. So, immediately thank Him for the healing you are about to receive.

When you pray for food, do you wait till you have eaten to pray? You shouldn't. The food is sanctified by the Word of God. So, you need to pray before you eat.

In the same way, you pray for your health, you are healed when you receive it. So, receive it as soon as you are prayed for, and see yourself healed. Walk in your healing. Give thanks for your healing.

> 1 Thessalonians 5:18 - in everything give thanks; for this is the will of God in Christ Jesus for you.

## May 8

God wants you well, He wants you totally healed, He wants your soul to live. People that go to hell lose their soul. The soul is your mind, your emotions, and your will. The mind and the emotions are still there, but they lose their will. They no longer have a choice.

Even in the Old Testament, through the prophets, God was telling people what to do so that they could be well, and they could live. In the verse below, Jeremiah was speaking to a king, but the words are true for anyone.

God has always wanted His people to be well, to live, and to join Him in heaven at the end of their life on earth. God loves people more than it seems possible. He loves you as much as He loves Jesus.

Praise God for His love, praise God for His healing, praise God for everything.

> Jeremiah 38:20 - ...Please, obey the voice of the LORD which I speak to you. So it shall be well with you, and your soul shall live.

## May 9

God is interested in you, you as an individual. He loves you as much as He loves Jesus, but your life, your thoughts, your plans, they are all of interest to God. If you are sick, have health issues, how much more effective could you be to God if you were healthy? He wants you well and healthy.

When God placed you on earth, He had plans for you. The best life you could ever have is to be in His perfect will. Hopefully, at times you are. That is when you will be the most productive, when you are in His perfect will.

This scripture says that He tests the mind. That word tests can be used to mean He tries, He checks, He wants to see if your mind, your thoughts, your plans are flowing in line with what He has for you to do.

When you are well, you can best witness to others. You can pray for others, you can be a testimony for God. When you are sick, you can do these things, but not as effectively. Learn to flow with God, to walk with Him, to be His witness.

> Jeremiah 17:10 - I, the LORD, search the heart, I test the mind, even to give every man according to his ways, according to the fruit of his doings.

## May 10

Israel did not always obey the instructions given to them by God. But the following is an excellent scripture to obey. Do you want all to be well with you? Obey the voice of God, be His child, and all will be well with you.

Learn to meditate scriptures, and trust God to show you how to walk in divine health. Also, share with others the things you learn so that others can have the same blessings you receive.

God has plenty for everyone. There is good health, good life, blessings for everyone. You don't need to horde the goodness of God. Share it and receive more. Learn to share, share testimonies, share things, share love.

Compassion for others is a part of love. Jesus healed all that were brought to Him because of the compassion He had for the sick. Seek the kingdom of God first, and learn to walk in compassion for others.

> Jeremiah 7:23 - But this is what I commanded them, saying, 'Obey My voice, and I will be your God, and you shall be My people. And walk in all the ways that I have commanded you, that it may be well with you.'

## May 11

Jesus suffered all sickness and all disease for you on the cross. He bore all with the stripes before He went to the cross. He suffered everything for your life on earth before the cross. He shed His blood for your total redemption.

He restored, He reconciled all things to Himself. He did all for you, which includes your total health. When sickness tries to come on you, stand up. Refuse it. It does not belong to you, it has no right to stay.

Do I make it sound easy? It is easy, but at times can seem very difficult. We have all prayed for, and with, many people who have spent weeks, months, and sometimes years claiming their victory. Don't quit, don't give in.

Jesus did not quit. He did not give in. Keep Him as your example, and realize that you are His representative, His witness on this earth. You have the authority in His name. Hold fast to that authority. The victory is yours.

> Colossians 1:20 - and by Him to reconcile all things to Himself, by Him, whether things on earth or things in heaven, having made peace through the blood of His cross.

## May 12

Who wants a sick heart? That does not always mean the physical heart, sometimes people refer to the spirit as the heart. That means the center of your soul, where your emotions are formed. You do not want that part of you sick either.

When your hope is blocked, when your hope is lost, your heart becomes sick. It may not be a physical sickness, but even emotional sickness is not good. God wants you well, spirit, soul and body.

When the hope is renewed, the desire comes, it is like a tree of life. You are revived. Your health returns. This can happen before the hope is actually met.

One example, if you are told you are being laid off, do you practically panic? All hope of pay checks are gone? What will you do? That is how you feel.

Then, you are told, "We got a big contract, your job is available, and you are getting a raise." All panic leaves, fear is gone, and you see in your mind your pay checks getting bigger. That becomes like a tree of life to you.

Proverbs 13:12 - Hope deferred makes the heart sick, but when the desire comes, it is a tree of life.

## May 13

When you are sick, a weapon has been formed against you. Can you agree with that? Satan has formed a weapon against you. If people talk about your sickness, this is judging in agreement with that weapon.

Recognize that your words are important. Every word is important. Do not speak against other people  You need to keep what you say in line with the Word of God. You need to only speak positive things about friends, or family, who are sick.

There is no need to repeat the negative things that doctors say. Your report needs to be that your friends are redeemed. God's Word says they are the healed, and you are saying so. It is so easy to want to repeat the negative you have heard. Don't.

God says NO weapon formed against you shall prosper. That sickness can NOT prosper. But it also says every tongue which rises against you, you shall condemn. Don't let your tongue be one formed against other people.

> Isaiah 54:17 - No weapon formed against you shall prosper, and every tongue which rises against you in judgment you shall condemn. This is the heritage of the servants of the LORD, and their righteousness is from Me," says the LORD.

## May 14

Many people slow down their healing with their tongue. Do you realize that? Some people even cause their sickness with their tongue. "I'm catching a cold." Why didn't you just let it run by? Why did you catch it?

Did you go to the doctor? Did you repeat the doctor's report to several people? If you repeated it to even one person, your tongue caused you to buy it. The words of your mouth are far more important than many people realize.

God created the world with the words of His mouth. This is the way humans are to function. Jesus stopped the storm when He was on the boat with the words of His mouth. Had Peter spoken to the storm, he could have stopped it.

This is the way you are to function. If you quote scripture, you can be more effective in areas such as your health. Your body responds to scripture, it is medicine to your body. Harness your tongue, learn to walk in divine health.

> Psalm 39:1 - I said, "I will guard my ways, lest I sin with my tongue; I will restrain my mouth with a muzzle, while the wicked are before me."

## May 15

Man keeps learning more and more. Man learned to fly. The airplane was developed. Man learned to cure many diseases. Penicillin was like a miracle when it was first developed. It has healed many people.

It seems like we keep learning more and more. However, each time something is developed, more problems crop up. Some of these are stopped quickly, some take more time. The Good News is, there is nothing that God cannot cure.

There is no problem that God cannot solve. Put your trust in God. He may lead you to a doctor, but then you will need to trust God to direct the doctor as he develops a solution for whatever is wrong with you.

Keep God as your source. Trust Him, and He will always come through. Do not ever be afraid of a sickness or disease. Do not question it being healed. All things are possible with God.

> Luke 18:27 - But He said, "The things which are impossible with men are possible with God."

## May 16

When you are hurting, you want help NOW. Is that right? You think, "Why do I have to wait for my healing? The price has already been paid, help!" Sickness can be painful. It can be very tiring.

Sometimes, all you want to do is rest and sleep. You know all that you need to be doing, why are you wasting time sleeping? You have no energy. You feel drained, tired, and have no strength.

There are times when you have to wait. Your body just slows down. It takes the body time to get itself back in shape. Why? With burn patients, this has been a real lesson that doctors have learned. Infections and other problems often arise.

God knows more than doctors. He has answers for us that doctors do not have. There is nothing wrong with using the scripture below! "Make haste to help me, O Lord." Learn to trust God, to lean on God. Watch God hasten your healing.

Psalm 38:22 - Make haste to help me, O Lord, my salvation!

## May 17

When you are standing for a healing, it is so necessary to keep your mind focused on God, the Word, as well as being healed. At that time, you do not want to be in confusion, anxiety, or stressed about your situation.

It would be great if all healings were instant! Sometimes they are. Sometimes they are in steps. Often, there is more than one thing going on in your body, so you are not even sure what the real problem is!

This is why, if you keep your mind on God, maintain your peace, then He can direct you and guide you in your prayers and your confessions. I have one area which is definitely taking longer to clear up than some others. That is probably true of many people.

How many diseases cause a fever, headache, and other aches and pains? Lots. Doctors need to be led by God when they prescribe medicine! So many things conflict, so many things have similar symptoms.

Learn to trust God, keep Him first, and let Him keep you in perfect peace as you are healed.

> Isaiah 26:3 - You will keep him in perfect peace, whose mind is stayed on You, because he trusts in You.

## May 18

Usually I use at least one scripture in praying for people. Many people do not realize how important scriptures are. The Bible has God's words in it. It is our life. Scriptures are a major key for our health. They are medicine to our body.

Scriptures are used to renew your mind. They point the way for you, they show you what God has for you. They are food for your spirit. This is why I suggest you not only use scriptures telling you God heals, but scriptures which paint a picture in your mind of you being healed.

God's Word is life and truth. To walk in divine health, it is necessary to know what God expects for you to be able to do. Let the Bible paint pictures in your mind. Let the Bible be your picture for your life.

Many people say, "Find yourself in the Bible." That is not always a straight forward way to do things. But, you can definitely find what God expects of everyone, and for everyone, in the Bible. That is how you learn to be a doer of the Word.

Mark 13:31 - Heaven and earth will pass away, but My Words will by no means pass away.

## May 19

Do you know anyone who has problems breathing? Today, often you see a person who has an oxygen tank with them. This is not an uncommon problem.

Breathing problems can be caused by many problems. Sometimes heart issues, lung issues, some illnesses can cause breathing problems. One is pneumonia. There are others.

No matter what the cause, if you are having problems breathing, you want breath. That alone is something to pray over. Finding the root problem, and praying over that is also useful.

Every knee must bow to the name of Jesus. You don't always have a name. But you are redeemed from all symptoms, all illnesses.

When you are meditating scriptures, it is good not only to use scriptures telling you that God heals you, but it is good to use scriptures showing you healed. The scripture below says, "God gives breath...." What a beautiful picture of healing for someone with breathing problems.

> Isaiah 42:5 - Thus says God the LORD, Who created the heavens and stretched them out, Who spread forth the earth and that which comes from it, Who gives breath to the people on it, and spirit to those who walk on it:

# May 20

God's Words, are they always with you? What He has told you gives you peace, health, and adds wisdom to your life. This makes it very important to always keep His Words in your mind, and in your speech. They are medicine to your flesh.

It is so important to learn what the Bible tells you, to learn the things that you are to do. Knowing scripture gives you the upper hand over your enemy. God's Words are light. The enemy functions in darkness. You only have one enemy. People are not your enemy.

When John the Baptist was beheaded, what did Jesus do? Did He go after the ruler that had John beheaded? No. Jesus did not consider Herad the Tetarch His enemy. The real enemy was Satan.

Jesus went to be alone, but people followed them. Jesus healed the sick. That was a stab at Satan. That is what was a blow to the real enemy.

Psalm 119:98 - You, through Your commandments, make me wiser than my enemies; for they are ever with me.

## May 21

God wants you well. He wants you healed. He wants His people healed so much that, when He took the people out of Egypt, there was not one feeble person among them. Everyone who had been sick was healed as they prepared to leave.

Talk to God. If you have a health problem, God will answer you. He says that He will hear. Don't be moved if the healing is not instant. Your body takes time to heal. Some things just naturally need time.

If you do not already know this, a good way to talk to God is by putting Him in remembrance to what His Word says. If you talk to Him with scriptures, you show Him that you have studied the Bible, and you know what is yours from the Bible.

When Jesus taught the people, He quoted Isaiah 61:1 as he started. He would use this and teach about healings and other things when He was ministering. (Luke 4:17-19)

If Jesus used scriptures, shouldn't you follow His example?

> Isaiah 65:24 - "It shall come to pass that before they call, I will answer; and while they are still speaking, I will hear.

## May 22

There is a form of prayer that has not been talked about a lot here. This is when you make a petition, or a prayer of supplication, to the Lord. These prayers are normally done in writing. Find the scriptures you are standing on, and make a formal request to God.

This needs to be written so that you have a record of what you are asking God for. You have the scriptures that you will quote daily written. Possibly, you will have someone agree with you over this prayer. If so, they will sign this also.

This is a very good and scriptural method of prayer. There are many scriptures telling you that God wants you well. Find the scriptures that address exactly what is your prayer. Put them in a petition.

Then, at least once a day, read the petition out loud. That reminds you of what is your goal. That feeds the scriptures into your spirit. The scriptures are medicine to your flesh. This keeps your mind fresh on your belief.

The scripture below tells you that this is a valid way to pray:

> 1 Kings 8:28 - Yet regard the prayer of Your servant and his supplication, O LORD my God, and listen to the cry and the prayer which Your servant is praying before You today:

## May 23

God desires you to be healthy. This is why He has promised healing, He has made healing available to everyone. It is a sign to the non-believer, it is available to the believer. Desire life, long life. Then you may see the goodness of God.

If you have long life, and goodness of days, witness to others. Pray for others. Watch others get healed as you pray for them. That blesses God when His children tell others how good God is.

There have been healing revivals in this world, and these are certainly years that God wants a healing revival going on. It has been prophesied. That makes it our job to pray and to take the steps to tell others what is available.

Don't be afraid. What if you pray and the person doesn't get well? First, you have to believe they will. Second, it may not be instant, don't tell God HOW He has to do things. Know that the healing has started when you prayed.

God is good. Trust God.

Psalm 34:12 - Who is the man who desires life, and loves many days, that he may see good?

## May 24

Do you feel that as you get older things aren't working well? You can keep your body in better shape than used to be realized. The Word heals, joy gives you strength, eating right and exercising do take good care of your body.

Paul acknowledges that the body perishes, or decays, but it does not mean that you can't keep going. People did not live as long years ago because man has learned more about the body, and how to take care of it.

The inward man, your spirit, is renewed daily. This is another reason that it is so important to stay in the Word. The Word is what feeds the spirit. It helps to renew the spirit.

There are more older people today than I think any generation before has ever known. Learn to be helpful to those elders. See to it that they also get their daily dose of the Word.

> 2 Corinthians 4:16 - Therefore we do not lose heart. Even though our outward man is perishing, yet the inward man is being renewed day by day.

## May 25

Have you noticed there seem to be new problems, new diseases, things which haven't happened before happening healthwise? Maybe you are involved in this same sort of a problem. Maybe doctors don't know what to advise you, or the medicine they want you to take has worse side effects than the disease.

None of this is a mystery to God. First of all, is your doctor a spirit-filled Christian? That would help, he would have the guidance of God available. No matter what the circumstances, you need to be praying for your doctor. The scripture below tells you that God reveals deep and secret things.

Use scriptures, use prayer, and trust God. If you wonder about changing doctors, ask God. He will lead you. God wants the best for you more than you do. He knows the best paths for you to follow. Let God lead you, praise Him, and follow His directions.

> Daniel 2:22 - He reveals deep and secret things; He knows what is in the darkness, and light dwells with Him.

## May 26

Walking in divine health, staying well, or getting well, are all conditions that should describe everyone. Some good advice for everyone is don't get angry. Anger, stress, frustration, all can lead to sickness. They are not good for your mind or your body.

What do you do when someone does you wrong? I have found there is one company that, every time I call them, I start tensing up. They are dishonest and causing me a problem. I have looked for alternatives. Talking to them does not accomplish anything.

In today's world, there seem to be a lot of situations where stress could take over. Learn to slow down. Speak blessings. Pray blessings over yourself. Keep telling yourself that blessings are chasing after you. This will lead to blessings.

Learn to think about the good when stressful situations arrive. Bring to your mind something good which has happened. Find scriptures telling you that you are blessed, quote those when you are in a potentially stressful situation.

As joy arises in you, strength will arise. This will help you to pull away from the stressful thoughts.

> Psalm 37:8 - Cease from anger, and forsake wrath; do not fret—it only causes harm.

## May 27

God formed you in the womb. He made you. If a person is born deformed, did God make them deformed? The answer is no. God does not do anything that is not perfect.

Many things can happen once the baby is conceived. Through foods the mother eats, chemicals in the environment, drugs she takes, many things can affect the baby. Drugs not only includes illegal drugs, but medicines. Many medicines have things which affect the unborn baby.

Some of these medicines are now known and no longer used. Many of the bad effects are still being learned.

If you have a Toyota, would you take it to a Ford dealership to be worked on? No. This shows why finding a Christian doctor helps, especially a spirit-filled doctor. Then the doctor can call upon God for help in treating you.

Seek God concerning your health. God wants you totally healed.

> Isaiah 44:24 - Thus says the LORD, your Redeemer, and He who formed you from the womb: "I am the LORD, who makes all things, Who stretches out the heavens all alone, Who spreads abroad the earth by Myself;

## May 28

Do you keep God first in your life? Do you keep God first in your mind? That is what is going to have to come first. Jesus told you to seek first the Kingdom of God. Don't you see, that includes keeping God first in your life?

Several ministers said they have had to give up some TV programs they were watching. Why would that be? Because those TV programs were pulling their mind to the world's way of thinking, away from God's way of thinking.

One of those ministers was telling that his daughter, about three years old, was sick. His prayers were not working. He realized that he had not kept God first.

When you want your healing, God is there, He is waiting, He wants you healed. Let God be first in your life. Don't complain to other members of the family, let them watch you and follow you.

In this scripture, when is "then"? It is when you are listening to God, and doing what He wants you to do.

> Jeremiah 29:12 - Then you will call upon Me and go and pray to Me, and I will listen to you.

## May 29

Healing is available to everyone. God has made provision for healing. For the non-believer, it is a sign to show them that Jesus is Lord. It is an invitation to bring them to Jesus as their Lord and Savior.

For the believer who will trust God, follow His directions, be a doer of the Word, it can be a matter of learning to walk in divine health. That is the best way to live. Just walk in good health.

There are times when the enemy sneaks in and lays something on you. God has given you everlasting strength. Trust God, meditate healing scriptures, and watch yourself be up and about, quickly.

Keep your thoughts focused on the fact that you are the healed. You are the victor. Keep your mouth speaking the positive. Do not yield to any other action.

> Isaiah 26:4 - Trust in the LORD forever, for in YAH, the LORD, is everlasting strength.

## May 30

People have more control over their bodies than most people realize. I have always hated having blood tests done. One time, a phlebotomist said to me, "You are not letting me have any blood." He explained I could stop the flow. I said, "Just a minute." I repented and I prayed. Immediately, the tube started filling.

There are many examples of people actually controlling some sickness in their body. Doctors know that someone's attitude can affect their healing. This is also used demonically. One report said that Voodoo deaths were caused mentally.

If you are bleeding, can you stop the flow of the blood? In the scripture below, Jesus healed this woman, but her belief that He could aided the healing. I know of one pastor who was in a dentist office and the dentist was trying to stop the flow of blood in his mouth. When the pastor found out the problem, he said, "Give me a minute." He prayed and the bleeding stopped.

Learn to take authority over your body. There are many areas where you can.

> Mark 5:29 - Immediately the fountain of her blood was dried up, and she felt in her body that she was healed of the affliction.

## May 31

One of the best things you can do to walk in good health, or to obtain a healing if you are sick, is to watch your mouth. Learn to speak the good. You can save your life by doing that. The scripture below tells you that.

Don't speak the bad. Don't tell everyone how bad you feel. If the doctors say there is no hope, keep that to yourself. Receive prayer, then know that you are healed. Speak what the Bible says. Let the weak say they are strong.

Is that lying? No. Lying is when you are deliberately deceiving someone. You are not trying to deceive anyone. You are calling those things which be not into being. You are speaking your faith. You are bringing the healing into existence.

Learn to guard your tongue, to be silent when you want to speak bad things. Do not use your tongue to talk about how bad the enemy is. Use your tongue to witness to others to tell of the goodness of God.

> Proverbs 13:3 - He who guards his mouth preserves his life, but he who opens wide his lips shall have destruction.

## June 1

The scripture below says that the lamp of the body is the eye. Does this mean if someone is blind they cannot be full of light? This is not actually talking about the physical eye. This is talking about the eye of the mind.

If your mind is full of scripture, if you have knowledge of the Bible, then your mind's eye is full of light. This means your whole body will be full of light. God is light. The enemy only operates in darkness. He can only operate where you have no knowledge.

This means you need knowledge of God's healing scriptures. If you do not know that Jesus paid the price for your healing with the stripes on His back, then you can not claim that for yourself or others.

If you don't know that ALL sickness and disease are under the curse of the law, and that you are redeemed from the curse of the law, then you cannot claim that for yourself and for others.

If you don't know that you have authority over sickness, then you can't claim that authority. Learn healing scriptures. Learn what you have.

> Matthew 6:22 - The lamp of the body is the eye. If therefore your eye is good, your whole body will be full of light.

## June 2

The 91st Psalm is good for walking in divine health. In verse 6, the word pestilence covers all sickness and all disease. It covers much more, but those are included in that word. Do not be afraid of them, you are redeemed from sickness and disease.

God wants you well, He wants you walking in divine health. Just reading that psalm every day can do much for you, your household, and all of your property. If you have a garden, think what it would do for your plants.

Learn to trust the Lord. He is your friend. He wants the best for you. God has given you so many tools to walk in divine health. Do not use these just for yourself. Use them for your family.

Learn to pray for others, teach others what you have learned about healing. Tell others that God wants them well.

> Psalm 91:5–6
> 5 You shall not be afraid of the terror by night, nor of the arrow that flies by day,
> 6 nor of the pestilence that walks in darkness, nor of the destruction that lays waste at noonday.

## June 3

When Jesus was on the earth, He did good and He healed all who were oppressed by the devil. He did this with the Holy Spirit and power. When you are born again, you receive the Holy Spirit. So, if you are born again, you can do the works that Jesus did.

There is an infilling of the Holy Spirit which gives you more, but every one who is born again has the Holy Spirit. Every Christian has the power in them that Jesus had in order to pray for people to be healed.

There is much more that can be done, there are other ways, but no Christian should feel that they can't pray for the sick and watch them recover. There are times when some evangelists have a greater anointing, but they are not always available.

If you need prayer, get a born-again friend to pray for you. If you know someone who is sick, pray for them. Use the ability you have in you.

> Acts 10:38 - how God anointed Jesus of Nazareth with the Holy Spirit and with power, who went about doing good and healing all who were oppressed by the devil, for God was with Him.

## June 4

If you are seeking healing, pray, believe and receive. There are times when you need more knowledge. There are times when you do not know what to pray for. There are times when wisdom is needed.

In the case of a ruptured appendix, the symptoms are the same as other problems. You may need to seek medical advice. At times, you will need to seek God for advice of where to go and what to do. Is this a time you need to go to the doctor?

Once you have knowledge, then you can seek God for the steps you need to take. Does this sound familiar? You need knowledge of the scriptures. There are times when you need knowledge of what is going on in your body.

God has given medical science help. There are times when He expects you to draw on the help from the doctors. When medical science does not have the answer, knock, ask God for more direction. Always pray for God to direct the doctor.

> Luke 11:9 - So I say to you, ask, and it will be given to you; seek, and you will find; knock, and it will be opened to you.

## June 5

All sickness and all disease comes from the evil one. God did not create any sickness or any disease. He wants His people whole and well. Don't ever forget those facts. Many scriptures tell you this.

God is interested in your health—spirit, soul, and body. He created the whole man, and He wants His man whole. God is faithful, He has established you. If you let Him, He will guard you from the evil one.

How do you block God from protecting you? One way is with the words of your mouth. If you speak things not in line with what the Bible says, you give place to darkness. That is what Job did. He spoke wrongly.

Learn to appreciate God, to spend time with God, to praise and worship Him. When you spend your time this way, you invite Him to guard you.

> 2 Thessalonians 3:3 - But the Lord is faithful, who will establish you and guard you from the evil one.

## June 6

Are you seeking healing? Is your health not up to par? Are you working on walking in divine health and you need help? The Holy Spirit is your helper. He will teach you all things. He can help you learn more about healing.

God does expect you to read the Bible, and to read healing scriptures. The Holy Spirit will bring to your remembrance all things. It is much easier to bring things to your remembrance if you have read them.

Will the Holy Spirit teach you things you have never heard or read? Probably. But once again, it is easier to help you when you have done your homework.

Develop your relationship with the Holy Spirit. If you are born again, you have the Holy Spirit in you. There is an infilling available which will increase your relationship. That is recommended.

> John 14:26 - But the Helper, the Holy Spirit, whom the Father will send in My name, He will teach you all things, and bring to your remembrance all things that I said to you.

## June 7

If you, or someone you know, is believing for a healing, there are some things that you need to do. First, you need to pray or have others pray for you. Once prayer has been done, healing needs to be received.

Healings can take time. Some are instant. If yours is not instant, you need to cast the burden of the healing on the Lord. It is not your burden, and it can wear you down. Burdens can become stressful and can be an anxiety. These will only make the situation worse.

Once you have received the healing, and once you cast the burden on the Lord, God will sustain you. As you meditate on healing scriptures (your medicine), the medicine is doing the work. You need to let God sustain you through this time.

Are you born again? Then you are the righteousness of Jesus. God will never let the righteous be moved, be hurt, be harmed. God will help you through the healing process and protect you.

> Psalm 55:22 - Cast your burden on the LORD, and He shall sustain you; He shall never permit the righteous to be moved.

## June 8

Prayer can be fun, it can also appear to be a time of testing and trial. That should not be the case. God has told us how to pray, and what we can pray about. Healing is one thing that has many scriptures to back it up.

Don't let your flesh get in the way. Don't let a doctor's report cause you to fear. Don't let feelings be your judge. As an act of your will, you need to trust God and stand on the Word.

Prayer that is based on scripture, with the scripture quoted, is always a good prayer. Find several healing scriptures, and feed them into your heart. Meditate on them, as you do this you will learn them.

Then, when you pray for yourself, or other people, out of the abundance of your heart you can pray. The scripture you have filled into your heart will come out in abundance. Healings will be available for yourself and others. If ever you are afraid, trust in God.

Psalm 56:3 - Whenever I am afraid,
I will trust in You.

## June 9

God wants you well. He wants you healed. He wants you living a long life. Learn to accept what God has for you. Learn what He expects of you to achieve a long life. If you will study, learn, and listen, you will live long.

God never designed man to be a temporary thing. First of all, the real you is a spirit, you have a soul, and your earth suit is a body. That body is not the body you will have for eternity.

God made the body out of dust on the earth. When you are on earth, you will have a body. So how do you take care of it? Take medication daily. What medication? Scriptures. Read them out loud. This way you are using your eyes to see the scripture, your ears to hear them, your mouth to speak them. You are also feeding your spirit and renewing your mind. Look at what a few minutes each day will do.

If there is sickness involved that you have already prayed over, take this medicine several times a day. Then God will protect you, even to your old age.

Isaiah 46:4 - Even to your old age, I am He, and even to gray hairs I will carry you! I have made, and I will bear; even I will carry, and will deliver you.

By Patricia L. Whipp

## June 10

Faith is needed for healing. There are times when people are healed by someone else's faith. For example, healing evangelists carry a strong healing anointing. They have maintained their faith for that blessing.

God expects you to develop your own faith. You can only be healed by someone else's faith a few times. One minister said he could pray for a family member once, then they had to start adding their faith to the prayer.

Faith comes by hearing. If you silently read a scripture, you are not hearing it. If you just listen to TV ministers, you may not be seeing the scripture. A deaf person can sign their scripture. They are using their body to build it into their heart.

A blind person can use braille, or they can use the Bible on CDs as well as listen to teaching.

Learn your Bible. Study your Bible.

Romans 10:17 - So then faith comes by hearing, and hearing by the Word of God.

## June 11

God's health plan is a great health plan. Jesus died, suffered beatings so you could be free from every sickness and disease that there ever has been or ever will be. What more could you ask for?

No matter where your health is today, excellent, or in the hospital dying, thank Jesus for what He has done for you. If you are in the hospital dying, there should only be two solutions; you go to heaven, or you get well. If you are not born again, receive Jesus as your Lord and Savior now.

God loves you with a love that is not understood. More and more is being learned by some people, but most people have no concept of the love of God. The fact that God loves you as much as He loves Jesus is also hard to accept.

Sing to the Lord. Sing praises to Him. Thank Him daily for what He has done for you. Seek first the Kingdom of God. Learn what He wants for you to do for Him.

Isaiah 12:5 - Sing to the LORD, for He has done excellent things; this is known in all the earth.

## June 12

God wants your health to be great. If you are born again, then your soul is delivered from death, from all evil after you leave this earth. God is merciful to you on this earth. All of us goof at times. Praise God for His mercy.

The verse below also means that your soul is delivered from evil here on earth as well. One translation says that you are pulled from the brink of disaster. Another says that you are rescued from death.

Walk in peace, walk in the presence of God. Keep yourself aware that God is in you. He wants the best for you. Don't do things you wouldn't do without God. This is why maintaining the awareness of God is so important.

God says He will guide your steps. He knows how to keep you in good health, He knows how to keep you in peace. Learn to listen, learn to follow the direction that you are supposed to go.

> Psalm 86:13 - For great is Your mercy toward me, and You have delivered my soul from the depths of Sheol.

## June 13

Have you ever watched a duck with ducklings? Have you seen the little ducklings crawl up on her back, under her wings? Looks crowded in there, but those little ducklings are safe from evil monsters that way. They are also safe from predators.

That is how much God loves you and wants you safe. He wants you safe from sickness, disease, and other predators. The devil is a predator. He would devour you just because you are God's child.

It is not normal human nature to trust another person totally. You may think you do, but deep down there is doubt, fear, questions. You are going to have to push past those doubts, to learn to trust God. God does not lie. What His Word says is true.

Meditate on these. Find scriptures which tell you this. It is so important to walk closely with God, to know He loves you, and to trust Him with your life. Your health may depend on your doing this. Your life may depend on this.

> Psalm 91:4 - He shall cover you with His feathers, and under His wings you shall take refuge; His truth shall be your shield and buckler.

## June 14

Are you believing for a healing? Do you want to pray for people who want to be healed? Both are great things to do. God wants you healed. He paid a tremendous price for the healing of people today.

Even in the Old Testament, God wanted people healed. He gave them very legalistic ways that they could go to the priests and obtain healing. I am sure that some people simply prayed the Psalms, and other scriptures, and were healed. All of this is also available today.

This psalm was written before Jesus, but we know that every knee must bow to the name of Jesus. You can use the name of Jesus, and any sickness must bow its knee. How easy is that?

These things just don't happen. You must believe. How do you do this? Feed these scriptures into your spirit. Meditate on scriptures, study the Word, see how things line up. As you study the Bible, the patterns are there. Trust God, and believe.

> Psalm 124:8 - Our help is in the name of the LORD, Who made heaven and earth.

## June 15

Are you believing for a healing, or praying with someone who is believing for a healing? Does the person who is believing for healing have unforgiveness? It is so important to walk in total forgiveness. If you see someone and you react in a negative manner, check with God, have you fully forgiven the person?

Anger, any kind of malice toward someone, can not only hinder your health, it will add to bad health. Those bad feelings will grow in you and will cause problems in you.

If you are afraid of someone, this is something to be dealt with. If there is spousal abuse, you need to seek God. Separation until things can be worked out may be necessary. If someone has threatened you, seek help. Do not stay in that situation.

The emotions, the hurts need to be dealt with. You don't need expensive help, there are agencies, places that help is available. Often, the church can offer help. This is not uncommon.

God loves you, He wants you well, He has help available.

> Ephesians 4:31 - Let all bitterness, wrath, anger, clamor, and evil speaking be put away from you, with all malice.

## June 16

When things have happened that cause you to be upset, hurt, distraught, you are opening the door for sickness. An example of this could be a broken marriage, or the loss of a child. Your life has changed and will probably never be the same.

I have seen, more than once, where the loss of a child caused a couple to separate and be divorced. This is a time for them to pull together. They need each other, they need to comfort each other.

Trauma may lead to mental illness, if not physical illness. Recognize that these things that cause such extreme hurts are from the devil. This can be a very difficult time to get a hold of your emotions, but that is what can help your life more than anything else.

Don't look to blame someone. If you need to forgive, that is the way to start recovery. It is not always easy, but once you make the decision and take the step, it becomes easier. Take the step.

When you are hurt, God is close to you at these times. Draw from God. Learn to think about other things, learn to put aside the hurts. Draw strength from God. Look for ways to experience joy. Let God's peace rise up in you.

Psalm 34:18 - The LORD is near to those who have a broken heart, and saves such as have a contrite spirit.

## June 17

Over and over in the Word you are told to take heed, to be a doer of the Word, to follow instructions in the Word of God. This applies to everyone. A part of walking in divine health means to learn to follow what you are told to do in the Bible.

Learning to walk in divine health, in other words to never be sick, should be the goal of everyone. Sickness is never from God, and certainly you do not want anything which is designed by the devil.

Steps to take to follow God involve, first of all, making a commitment to God. Receive Jesus as your Lord and Savior. Tell God you love Him, and want to serve Him. Read His Word. Listen to teachers, today there are many excellent choices.

Then walk the walk, talk the talk that you are learning. Seek first the Kingdom of God, that is a good path to cleanse your way.

> Psalm 119:9 - How can a young man cleanse his way? By taking heed according to Your Word.

## June 18

God formed you in the womb. God created man, and has formed all humans since then. He has named you. He has called you by your name. If He tells Jacob and Israel to "Fear not," don't you think He says the same thing to you?

God loves all of His children. He wants you healthy, He wants you whole. There are no physical problems which He cannot overcome. There is no disease, no sickness, for which God has not provided healing. Learn to trust God.

Find scriptures that tell you His promises. Use those scriptures as a vaccine when you are healthy, and as medicine when you are sick.

Remember, God loves you.

Isaiah 43:1 - But now, thus says the LORD, who created you, O Jacob, and He who formed you, O Israel: "Fear not, for I have redeemed you; I have called you by your name; you are Mine!

## June 19

When God tells you that you can have life, that does not mean a sick, uncomfortable, miserable life. That means healthy, active, lively, strong life. That is what God considers life. Look at the definitions of the Hebrew and Greek words to see that.

By humility, that does not mean being bent over, afraid to speak, thinking everyone else is better than you. That means being submitted to God. A humble person is someone who is submitted to God

By the fear of the Lord, that does not mean being afraid of God. That means a reverence, a total reverence for God; a reverence for who God is, for what He does, for the power He has; a reverence for what He has done, what He does, and what He is going to do.

Out of humility and fear, or reverence of God, are riches, honor, and life. Think of those. Be sure you are submitted to God, be sure you trust God, be sure you love God. Tell Him all of these. Tell Him you love Him, and thank Him for His love for you.

Proverbs 22:4 - By humility and the fear of the LORD are riches and honor and life.

171

# June 20

Learn to listen. Don't listen to the noise of the world. Don't listen to the complaints of others, learn to listen for the Holy Spirit. He will guide you, He will show you the path to walk. He will guide you down the path for divine health.

God wants you doing things for Him. Yes, He is interested in your life, but if you line your life up to what He wants for you, it will be best. Today, everyone seems to try to be doing everything, and they are not discerning what is best for them.

Learn to seek God. As you plan events for your children, seek God. Let Him guide you. The health of your whole family can improve if you do this. Your health as well. Is every sport necessary? Maybe it is, but if it is at the expense of church, you might reconsider.

God is interested in every part of your life, not just church. God is interested in where you live, who you fellowship with, how you dress, everything. Start including God in things that you have not before. Watch what He will do for you.

Proverbs 15:31 - The ear that hears the rebukes of life will abide among the wise.

## June 21

What does irrevocable mean? It means that something cannot be changed. Once it is placed or accepted, it stands forever. Healing is a gift from God. He has stated that healing is available to anyone who wants it. There are things which must be done, it is not automatic, but it is available.

This is another way of saying that God's Word cannot fail. God cannot lie. Sometimes you have done everything right. Your body is working on the healing, maybe the angels are bringing a new body part, everything is fine, time is needed.

What do you do? Keep up your confession, "I am healed of...." Keep reading the healing scriptures out loud. They are renewing your mind, they are medicine to your body, they are feeding your spirit. They are keeping the angels moving if they are involved.

God cannot fail. If you quit, if you change your confession, then you can refuse your healing. Stay committed. Know that it is on it's way.

Romans 11:29 - For the gifts and the calling of God are irrevocable.

## June 22

God heals you in many ways. Often, we do not realize that we have been healed. At an afterglow meeting one evening, a young man was sitting on the floor. When he had arrived at the meeting, he was going in for knee surgery the next day.

A lady at the meeting said, "Could you have sat like that when you came in here?" He was in total shock. He said, "No," he realized his knee was healed. When pain comes on, it makes itself known. As it leaves, often that is not noticed.

Using the Word, meditating on it, listening to it on a regular basis, helps give opportunity for these healings to take place. Many times I have realized that a pain I had been experiencing has gone.

Give thanks to God. Praise Him for these miraculous healings. Pray for others, pray for the move of the spirit throughout the world, that there will be many of these things taking place in the days ahead.

> Psalm 107:1 - Oh, give thanks to the LORD, for He is good! For His mercy endures forever.

## June 23

Comfort others. Help build up other people. When someone is sick, when they don't feel well, they need to be built up. If someone is standing for a healing, just reading healing scriptures to them can be an encouragement.

When someone's faith is stretched thin, just visiting them can be a boost up. It can help them get through the next few hours to the next few days. Sometimes, talking to someone on the phone can be an encouragement.

If you have studied the Bible, meditated on scriptures, the Holy Spirit has something to help you say to others. You have built into your spirit things which He can use to build others up. This does not just have to be people who are sick, anyone.

Learn to have a word of encouragement ready.

> 1 Thessalonians 5:11 - Therefore comfort each other and edify one another, just as you also are doing.

## June 24

Be a doer of the Word daily for healing. Meditate healing scriptures. If you and everyone you know are walking in divine health, praise God for that. If you have prayed for healing, praise God for your healing.

There are people who are sick. Pray for healing revivals in America. That is a sign and wonder to the unsaved.

Learn to watch your mouth. Speak words of wisdom to yourself and others. This is true not just for healing, this is true in every area of your life. This is a good way to live, both at home and in a business environment.

As you do this, as you meditate in scriptures, as you speak wisdom, you will have understanding in your heart. This means that you will have help, knowledge of what to do. If you are looking for help with a healing, it could come there. If you are at work wondering how to solve a problem, it could be there.

Your words control your life far more than most people understand.

Psalm 49:3 - My mouth shall speak wisdom, and the meditation of my heart shall give understanding.

# June 25

Do you stick close to God? Learn to do that. God is always there for you. He will help you, He will uphold you. If you were to stumble, God would be there to stop you from falling.

One time, there was something very slippery, soap or grease, on my kitchen floor. I stepped on it, and literally 'slid' upright across the kitchen to the counter. I realized that, without divine help, I would have been flat on the floor.

There are many things which can cause someone to fall. Often, when people are sick, they will feel dizzy. They might find it hard to walk. This happens with vertigo, but there are other times that people can have dizzy problems as well.

God will uphold you. He will protect you. Sometimes, an angel protects you from falling. Learn to walk closely with God. Let Him protect you.

> Psalm 63:8 - My soul follows close behind You; Your right hand upholds me.

## June 26

God wants you healed. He has always wanted His people healed. Hezekiah, the leader, was dying. Isaiah went to see Hezekiah to set his house in order, he was going to die. As Isaiah left, Hezekiah turned his face to the wall and prayed.

God stopped Isaiah as he was leaving. He told Isaiah to go back to Hezekiah and tell him that he would live fifteen more years. On the third day, he was to go to the house of the Lord.

That was a covenant partner, not a son or daughter. If God listened to people from the Old Testament, how much more do you think a son or daughter who is walking in faith will receive God's attention?

God loves you with an everlasting love. He wants you well, He wants you healed. Plead your case, find your scriptures, and watch what God will do for you.

> 2 Kings 20:5 - "Return and tell Hezekiah the leader of My people, 'Thus says the LORD, the God of David your father: "I have heard your prayer, I have seen your tears; surely I will heal you. On the third day you shall go up to the house of the LORD.

## June 27

If you are fighting a sickness, you are fighting against the devil. He is the one who brings all sickness and disease. One of the ways to fight this is with the name of Jesus. You have authority over all sickness and disease.

Through the name of Jesus, you take this authority. As you push against the enemies of God, through the name of Jesus, you will trample down the ones who try to rise against you, all of those who rise up against you.

God has done so much for you, and for your healing. He sent Jesus to the cross. Jesus bore all of your illness, pain, grief, as well as all of your sin before, on, and after the cross. The price for your divine health has been paid.

There may be times when you have to take an active stand, but never forget the tools you have been given, that the price has been paid, and you are the victor.

> Psalm 44:5 - Through You we will push down our enemies; through Your name we will trample those who rise up against us.

## June 28

When you are sick, often you feel weak. You need strength. God is with you. He will strengthen you. In fact, He will heal you. God wants you healed more than you do. He paid a tremendous price for your healing. His Son, Jesus, was sent to the cross, and was beaten before going to the cross for your healing.

Many people don't realize that healing is available. You have to apply your faith. God often heals the unsaved as a sign that He is. But God expects the Christian to start using their faith. You can be healed by faith healers, but then you need to start applying your faith.

Once you are healed, use your faith to stay healed. Then, learn to start walking in divine health. Then, you do not need healing. Also, God will hold you up with His hand. Learn to walk as God intended man to be when He made Adam.

> Isaiah 41:10 - Fear not, for I am with you; be not dismayed, for I am your God. I will strengthen you, yes, I will help you, I will uphold you with My righteous right hand.'

## June 29

Are you believing for a healing which you have received? They don't always manifest instantly. Some things take time. A broken bone takes time in the natural for it to mend, and sometimes it takes time in the spiritual world.

What you need to do as you are believing for the manifestation is to dig into the Word of God. Learn more about what the Bible says about healings. Learn to live in God, and God's Word, and let God's Word live in you.

This is true of many things, not just healing. However, it is excellent advice for healing. After a healing manifests, you need to stay in the Word to maintain your healing. I witnessed one lady in a healing line who kept saying, "I don't believe it." As she kept saying that, the wound opened back up and started bleeding again.

Keep your words in agreement with the Bible, let God's Word be alive in you, ask what you desire, and it shall be done for you.

> John 15:7 - If you abide in Me, and My words abide in you, you will ask what you desire, and it shall be done for you.

By Patricia L. Whipp

# June 30

If you, or someone in your family, has what the doctors call an incurable disease, it can be like a mountain. It can control the home, definitely the atmosphere of the home. If the person is not functional, then everyone else at one time or another is usually involved.

Some examples would be final stages of cancer; extreme cases of Alzheimer's; a child born with a problem that the child can never function on their own. These can all become a weight, a mountain in your life.

Every one of these problems is something which can be healed. God wants the person healed, He wants them set free. Other members of the family need to agree and set their faith. If the person can join in, great.

It would be helpful to take the person to a place where healings are occurring, such as Healing School at Rhema, Eagle Mountain International Church services, Richard Robert's services, to name a few. There are others.

Don't give up, don't loose faith. Trust God, and watch the mountain be cast into the sea.

> Mark 11:23 - For assuredly, I say to you, whoever says to this mountain, 'Be removed and be cast into the sea,' and does not doubt in his heart, but believes that those things he says will be done, he will have whatever he says.

## July 1

Have you ever heard that, if you pray for something twice, it will be negated and you will not receive it?  That depends on your heart attitude.  If you are praying a second time because you think you weren't heard the first, there might be truth to that.

If you are praying something like the Lord's prayer, or the Ephesians prayer, where you are reading scriptures, and you are praying for more, or deeper help, you are basically meditating the Word which is what  Joshua 1:8 tells you to do.

Often, with a sickness, new problems can arise.  Daily, there are new things that you can combat.  Especially when your prayer is mainly scripture, then go for it.  You are feeding more medicine into your body.  The scripture below tells you to keep on.

What you need to watch is your heart attitude.  Do not let doubt in, do not let fear in. Know that the victory is yours.  For example, if you are believing for a new knee joint, you are feeding your angels when you read scriptures. You are feeding your faith, you are keeping your mind alive with a picture of the finished healing. Go for it.

> Matthew 7:7 - "Ask, and it will be given to you; seek, and you will find; knock, and it will be opened to you.

## July 2

Sometimes, you know there is a health problem, but you don't know what to pray. There may be a spot on someone's body that does not look normal. There may be a balance issue, but no idea what is the problem. Worse yet, at times, the doctor does not know.

There are times when you need wisdom to know what to pray. Many people pray for the "unknown," and that may be what is needed. But God will give you wisdom, He will help you. Seek God for guidance over what to pray.

Often, friends and strangers judge your problem based on problems they have had. Because I have used a cane and a walker, the past few years people rush up to me, even on a street corner, and say, "You need to get hip surgery. It did wonders for me." My hips are fine.

God will help you with direction for your prayer, and with direction for scriptures to meditate. Pray and ask God for these. Then use them as you receive any direction. You may need to do this more than once. Probably, you will get one or two suggestions the first time, more later. Be consistent, and receive the victory.

> James 1:5 - If any of you lacks wisdom, let him ask of God, who gives to all liberally and without reproach, and it will be given to him.

# July 3

The verse below is for someone who is pregnant, or would like to be pregnant. It shows you that God wants you to have children. He wants your children to be blessed, which means to be healthy. God does not cause sickness.

God is good, everything which He does is good. People today are blaming God for so many problems, He is not the author of the bad that is in the world today. When Adam sinned, he turned control of earth over to the devil. Many problems are the fault of the devil.

Your flesh can cause you problems. Your flesh desires things that are not good for it, and that is a real problem for many people. Addictions, eating wrong things, these can all be problems of the flesh.

Learn to trust God. Learn to lean on God, listen to the spirit, and follow what God has for you. This includes children if you want children.

> Deuteronomy 28:4 - "Blessed shall be the fruit of your body, the produce of your ground and the increase of your herds, the increase of your cattle and the offspring of your flocks.

## July 4

Are you a disciple of Jesus? Of course, first you need to be born again. Then, you need to decide you truly want to be a disciple. You want to learn what the Word says, and you want to be a doer of the Word! Then you are a disciple.

You are free! You are free from sickness and disease. You have learned the keys, you should be applying your faith. This gives you light, it gives you knowledge that Jesus gave His body for your health.

The enemy operates in darkness. Once you have light, you have knowledge, you have authority over all areas of the enemy. Some things may take time to obtain your freedom, but it is available. Don't quit.

Start praising God for your freedom. Praise Him for what He has done for you.

> John 8:31–32
> 31 ..."If you abide in My word, you are My disciples indeed.
> 32 And you shall know the truth, and the truth shall make you free."

## July 5

God is always available for you to call on Him. He will answer. He will strengthen you, He will heal you. He has always had mercy on you. Learn to draw from God. Learn to trust Him. He will help you.

God's love for you is very evident in the things He has done. He gave His only son, He sent Jesus to earth for you. Jesus went to the cross for you. He went into hell and took the keys from Satan.

God heals. He has healed man from Genesis up to today. He is not going to stop today. He will always heal man as long as man needs healing. What steps do you need to take towards your healing?

You need to learn scriptures. You shouldn't believe something just because you heard someone say it. You need to know for yourself what the Bible says. You need to know that you have authority.

When you have scriptures behind you, when you know you have authority, then you can take the steps God has told you to take. Then, healing is yours.

> Psalm 6:2 - Have mercy on me, O LORD, for I am weak; O LORD, heal me, for my bones are troubled.

## July 6

Have you done something wrong? You have repented, but you believe you are not getting well because of what you did. This scripture is talking about the backslider. God says, "…I will heal him."

God always forgives. In fact, He forgets what you have done. You need to do the same thing. Learn to receive forgiveness. Then receive your healing. God wants everyone healed. He never makes anyone sick, He does not delay healing.

Healings often take time. That is because of the way the body works. That is not because God deliberately delays. It would take a miracle to make a healing be fast. Yes, God does miracles, but not always.

Backsliders are always welcome back. Take a look at the story of the prodigal son. (Luke 15:11-32) The father was looking daily for his son. He hastened to bring his son back. How much more does the Father God look for His backslidden child. He wants His backslidden child home, healthy, and fed.

> Isaiah 57:19 - "I create the fruit of the lips: peace, peace to him who is far off and to him who is near," says the LORD, "and I will heal him."

## July 7

God has always wanted His people well. God also has always healed His people. In Isaiah, it tells that He will strike Egypt, and heal it. It says the people will return to God and He will heal them.

In the Old Testament, they were under the law. There were laws about how everything was to be done. Man could not keep the law. Praise God that man does not have to try to keep the law now.

God had mercy on people in the Old Testament. Over and over He showed His mercy. He didn't rule by law, He often used His mercy. Today, in the New Testament, we have a much clearer way to obtain healing. But God still shows us a lot of mercy.

We have the right to claim healing, to get prayed for at church, or to take authority over all sickness and disease. The age in which we live has changed, but God has never changed. He often shows mercy to us, and He wants us healed.

> Isaiah 19:22 - And the LORD will strike Egypt, He will strike and heal it; they will return to the LORD, and He will be entreated by them and heal them.

# July 8

Everyone will die once, or be raptured. That is a fact. There is a time to heal, and a time to die. But, you don't have to be sick to die. Because I talk about healing, I had one lady think I must be afraid to die. No, to be absent from the body is to be present with the Lord.

There are people in the Bible who laid down and yielded up the spirit. I have heard of many who have done that during my life time. Lining up Solomon's writing with other scripture, now is always a time to heal.

God wants His people healed while they are on earth. He has made too much provision in the New Testament for healing to expect that you must be sick at times. Healing is God's best. Go for the best.

> Ecclesiastes 3:2–3
> 2 A time to be born, and a time to die; a time to plant, and a time to pluck what is planted;
> 3 a time to kill, and a time to heal; a time to break down, and a time to build up;

# July 9

Are you bold to speak out to other people about the Name of Jesus? Are you bold to offer to pray for someone to be healed? Peter and John were both told by the authorities they were not to speak out in the Name of Jesus. The scriptures below are their prayer for boldness.

Use this prayer. Speak up. Do not be fearful, you have God backing you up. He wants you talking about His Son. Just as Peter and John did, He wants you to develop a boldness within you to speak up.

It doesn't hurt to ask a few questions first. If you don't have a witness on what to say, finding out where people stand so you know what direction to go is not wrong, but speak up. Do witness. Offer to pray.

Meditating the scripture below could be a help to you to develop your boldness. Push yourself if necessary. Look for opportunities to witness, to pray for others for healing.

> Acts 4:29–30
> 29 Now, Lord, look on their threats, and grant to Your servants that with all boldness they may speak Your word,
> 30 by stretching out Your hand to heal, and that signs and wonders may be done through the name of Your holy Servant Jesus."

By Patricia L. Whipp

## July 10

God is good. He has planned healing for you from before the foundation of the world. Healing is a gift from God. Don't ever doubt that God wants you well. God does not have sickness to give you! God wants you totally healed.

It is so important to believe the Bible. There are people who, because of their life's experiences, say that the Bible is not true. Some have said that God put sick people here to teach us to love them. You will not find that in the Bible. Pray for those people.

Learn to love everyone, but do not be influenced by words that do not line up with the Bible. Just let those words go in your mind and out the other side. This is why so many movies and stories that are cute, funny, or sad, speak to your emotions, but can cause you to doubt God.

Learn to put God first, to only believe the Word, to trust God's love for you. A loving Father wants his children to be healthy, wise, and to have a good life. That is God's best, and that is His desire for His children.

> Psalm 117:2 - For His merciful kindness is great toward us, and the truth of the LORD endures forever. Praise the LORD!

# July 11

Healing is so important. There are times when you hurt, and you don't know what the problem is. You need help, but words escape you. God hears. God is concerned. God wants the best for you. When healing is needed, He wants to get it to you.

There are times when doing something the right way is needed, but there are times when just yelling, "Help," to God is enough. You can listen to many preachers. Most of the ones in the Word of Faith camp are saying the same thing, but sometimes they suggest different applications.

Lay out your problems to God. Try to find scriptures that support what you need. Then go to God with your request. Maybe you need wisdom. Maybe it isn't healing. One lady found that what she was wearing to sleep in had a snap on it which was rubbing and causing the sore she had. Wisdom says change your bed clothes.

There is no problem too small to go to God with, or too big. He wants the best for you, and can get answers to you.

> Psalm 140:6 - I said to the LORD: "You are my God; hear the voice of my supplications, O LORD.

## July 12

Where does all sickness come from? Is there sickness in heaven? There is no sickness in heaven. Until the fall, until Adam ate the forbidden fruit, there was no sickness. Sickness is designed and devised by the devil.

You have been given armor to protect yourself. Have you ever considered that using your armor will help you to maintain divine health? Your whole body is protected when you have on all of your armor. How could sickness get in if you have your armor on?

Truth, this is the belt. This not only covers your waist, but it holds all of the rest of the armor in place. Be sure to always walk in truth. By the way, the Word of God is truth.

Righteousness, this is your breastplate. Your feet are covered with the gospel. When you use your faith, that covers the front of you. That is your shield. Being born again is your helmet. Your head is covered.

The sword is a weapon, the sword is the Word of God. When you quote scriptures to the devil, you are slashing him with a sword. Prayer is also a weapon. Letting the spirit pray through you stops the devil in his tracks.

Maintain your armor.

Ephesians 6:11 - Put on the whole armor of God, that you may be able to stand against the wiles of the devil.

# July 13

People have been criticized for speaking their faith. Mainly this has been involved with healing. Someone is limping, and they say, "I am healed." If they have been prayed for, and they have received their healing, then they are healed.

At times, you need to just speak your faith. However, rather than cause people to think you are crazy, you can say something like, "By the stripes of Jesus, I am healed." You are still speaking the truth. There are times when this can be used, and it gives you an opening to witness.

It is very important to speak what the Bible says, but it is equally important to lead non-believers to Jesus. Non-believing Christians are babies. They also need to be led to the truth of what the Bible says.

Be gentle with how you talk to people. It is better to keep a bridge between yourself and others so that you can communicate. Building a wall between you and others is not productive.

> Colossians 4:6 - Let your speech always be with grace, seasoned with salt, that you may know how you ought to answer each one.

# July 14

Do you walk in love toward others? What does that have to do with healing? If you are not walking in love, then most likely you are getting into stress, you are not in peace, and you are having emotional problems.

All of these issues can lead to health issues. So, it looks like learning to walk in love is a key to divine health. Walking in divine health is where you should want to be walking. Start walking in love toward your fellow man.

Paul says in the scripture that walking in love is the bond of perfection. He probably was not thinking of your health when he wrote that, but it makes sense that it helps you to walk in divine health.

The scripture below says above all these things—if you look back at what people have done to you, if you remember offenses people have caused you, you are not walking in forgiveness. You are not walking the love walk.

Unforgiveness can cause more problems than most people realize. It is very bad on you in many ways. Ask God to show you anywhere that you are not in forgiveness. So, if your health is not good, I ask you, is your walking in love life good?

> Colossians 3:14 - But above all these things put on love, which is the bond of perfection.

# July 15

Sickness and disease did not exist before the fall of Adam. While Adam and Eve walked with God, light reigned in the earth. There was no sickness or any disease. After the fall, darkness came. Darkness is where the devil reigns.

When Jesus was raised from the dead, God delivered us from the power of darkness, He moved us into the kingdom of Jesus. Where are you walking? You have the right to walk healed. You have the right to be free from the powers of darkness.

Many people miss the fact that they are in a war. Because God has moved us into the kingdom, because we are delivered from the power of darkness, doesn't mean that you don't have to do anything. The devil does all he can to steal the Word from you.

If the devil can make you forget that you are redeemed from darkness, he will keep you in darkness. You have to keep the Word first in your mind, you have to remind the evil one of the fact that you are redeemed.

You do this with the Word. Quote the Word to the devil. It is like a sword, it slashes him. But you have to use the sword. God does not do it for you. That is your job.

> Colossians 1:13 - He has delivered us from the power of darkness and conveyed us into the kingdom of the Son of His love,

# July 16

Are you praying for healing? God answers prayer, and He delights in His people being healed. If you are making a supplication to God for anything, it is best to use scriptures. He told you to put Him in remembrance. Writing your prayer is also good.

Once you have your prayer the way you want it, pray it. Speak it to God. If it is in writing, read it to God. Putting it in writing is not for God, it is for you. You can then go back and remind yourself what you prayed.

Use the scriptures you selected to meditate. Saying them out loud daily is good. It has many benefits. The scriptures are medicine to your body, so as you read them, you are taking your medicine.

The scriptures also renew your mind so that you remember what you have prayed. As you do this, you should see yourself healed. Even when the healing is complete, doing this periodically keeps your healing maintained. Otherwise, the devil will try to steal the Word from you, and bring the sickness back.

Psalm 116:1 - I love the LORD, because He has heard my voice and my supplications.

## July 17

When you are upset, angry, hurt, and many other negative emotions, have you been told to 'vent'? Get it out, scream, hit a pillow, and many other ways of dealing with those negative feelings. Stop. You are taking those feelings on when you do that.

The most effective way to deal with those negative feelings is to turn to God. If you need to forgive someone, do that immediately. Grief is another area that the devil will use to rob you of life.

When you vent, you can cause mental anguish, depression, and other forms of problems which are not healthy. God wants you healthy. He wants every part of you healthy—physically, mentally, and spiritually. He wants you to be in good health.

Venting, in ways described above, are all things that the world has come up with for you to deal with these problems. God has better ways. Don't suppress feelings, deal with them. Forgive where necessary. Learn to ignore some of these feelings. Learn to turn to joy, and let joy be your strength to get you out of these feelings. Learn to maintain your joy, and maintain your peace.

Proverbs 29:11 - A fool vents all his feelings, but a wise man holds them back.

## July 18

Search God's Word. Find scriptures which tell you that God heals. Find scriptures which tell you that God wants you healed. There are many scriptures with these promises from God. God tells you to put Him in remembrance of His Word.

In the scripture below, God has shown Jeremiah something which He is going to do. God always performs His Word. There are many scriptures that tell us that God's Word will not return void.

God cannot lie. Many scriptures tell you that. His Word is true, and it is alive. He has promised you healing. He has promised you health. Know that God never fails. If you do not give up and quit, God's healings are available.

Whatever you have prayed for, pray in faith, believe, and receive. Know that it is yours. Speak the Word over it to water it, speak the Word over it to develop it. Watch the Word come to pass

> Jeremiah 1:12 - Then the LORD said to me, "You have seen well, for I am ready to perform My Word."

## July 19

Do you have problems walking? This could be because of problems with your feet, your knees, hips, any body part. It could be because you are so weak, your strength is gone due to an illness.

Trust God for His help for your healing. God wants you healed, He wants you well. He will make your paths straight for your feet. If the path were rough, possibly something could become dislocated. That would be even worse.

Learn to trust God. Don't expect God to prove Himself to you! God is faithful, He loves you. He sent His Son to earth for you. Don't even think, "If God will do this, then I will trust Him."

As an act of your will, set your mind to trust God. Learn to believe His Word. As you do these things, you will see your healing.

> Hebrews 12:13 - and make straight paths for your feet, so that what is lame may not be dislocated, but rather be healed.

## July 20

Are you praying for healing for yourself, or for someone else? It does not matter who is being prayed over. All sickness and disease are from the devil. God does not have any of that. You are of God, and you have already overcome anything that the evil one has!

This should strengthen your faith. You use your faith for healing. Knowing that you have overcome should add to your faith. Jesus paid the price for your healing, that should add to your faith.

There are so many scriptures that you could use here. This is one that is not often used for healing, but it applies. It is very strongly worded. The greater one is in you. Remind yourself of that at times.

Build up the picture, see the greater One in you. Know that you are the overcomer, apply that to healing, for yourself, and for others. Know that when you speak to a mountain, it must move. Why? Because the greater One is in you.

> 1 John 4:4 - You are of God, little children, and have overcome them, because He who is in you is greater than he who is in the world.

# July 21

When you are praying for healing, focus on Jesus. Focus on the revelation of what Jesus did for you. Place your hope fully on what Jesus did for you as He went to the cross. Recognize that all sickness and disease was placed on Him as He went to hell for you.

When you pray, your faith is the substance of what you hope for. (Hebrews 11:1) It means that, what you believe, what you are seeing, is real, and that you have every right to expect it to come to pass.

This is why it is so important to learn what is promised to you in the scriptures. If you are praying without the backing of the Bible, good luck. You are no longer relying on faith, you no longer have proof.

When you go to court, a lawyer finds laws saying that you have legal rights to what you are suing over. In the same way, your Bible is your proof that you have rights to what you are praying about. With healing, your Bible has proof that you have rights to be healed.

Get these scriptures built so strongly into you that you don't have to think about them. Learn to lean on the Holy Spirit to guide you.

> 1 Peter 1:13 - Therefore gird up the loins of your mind, be sober, and rest your hope fully upon the grace that is to be brought to you at the revelation of Jesus Christ;

By Patricia L. Whipp

## July 22

You want to learn God's ways. You want to learn what God expects of you. It is well known that God expects you to use faith. He gave you the measure of faith. You need to exercise that, so that it grows.

What else does God expect of you? He expects you to meditate His Word. He tells you that many places. There is much in the Bible that tells you that God wants you well. The fact that Jesus suffered all sickness and disease for you, that alone tells you that God wants you healed.

Healing is definitely one reason you need to learn what the Word says. This is one reason you need to study the Bible, to learn what steps you need to take to walk in divine health, and how you need to pray for others.

Once you have learned one thing, don't forget what you learned there as you move to the next thing. Many steps which you learn can be applied to healing, but they can also be applied to other areas of your life.

The Bible teaches principles which apply to every area of your life. Let the Holy Spirit guide you and teach you these things.

> Psalm 119:33 - Teach me, O LORD, the way of Your statutes, and I shall keep it to the end.

# July 23

God has everything for you, if you will let Him. He is your light, He is your salvation. That word for salvation carries many meanings. Being healthy is certainly a part of salvation, being wealthy, having eternal life are all a part of salvation.

Not everyone is healed when they are born again. Not everyone is made wealthy, but these are both available. Everyone does have eternal life when they are born again.

Let's look at the healthy side. If you have received Jesus, you have authority over all power of the enemy. You have nothing to be afraid of. God is the strength of your life. Often people who are sick feel weak. God is your strength. Draw on that strength. Do not be afraid. Many people fear illness.

There are so many ads on TV showing sickness, that pretty soon you begin to feel sick. Don't believe all the ads you see. Don't believe all that you hear. Seek God, the Word, and believe what the Word says!

There is nothing wrong with having a physical check-up, but use scriptures as vaccines to keep you healthy.

> Psalm 27:1 - The LORD is my light and my salvation; whom shall I fear? The LORD is the strength of my life; of whom shall I be afraid?

## July 24

From Genesis to Revelation, the Bible tells us of the goodness of God, the mercy of God, the consistency of God. We know that God never lies, everything He says is truth, and everything prophesied will come to pass.

This is true of healing. You do not have a new disease that God can't or won't heal. Constantly, new things are being found, some are being developed as a weapon, a type of warfare. Guess what? God is on top of it. He knows the cure. He knows how to restore your body to it's original design.

God does not use sickness to teach you things. Sickness is from the devil, and the devil is not your teacher. I do know people who believe that he is. If you are learning from the devil, drop him, let the Holy Spirit be your teacher.

Read the Bible, study the Bible, learn what it says. Do not let your experiences make the Bible untrue to you. The Bible is true. I can't stress this enough. God sent the Holy Spirit to teach you. If you are learning things that do not line up with the Bible, you had better check who you are learning them from.

God loves you, He is faithful, He is honest, He wants to bless you, He wants you whole.

Psalm 119:160 - The entirety of Your Word is truth, and every one of Your righteous judgments endures forever.

## July 25

The following scripture was said by Job. This is a statement made by Job which we can use, this is good. Unfortunately, Job did not do what he says that he did. That is part of what caused Job's problems.

Learn what are the commandments, or Words of God. Treasure His Words, treasure the Bible more than your food. That will help keep you well. Do you have problems with your stomach, or your digestive system? Part of the problem may be what you are saying.

Praying over your food is also very important. You don't want your food spoiled, or causing you problems. When it is sanctified by the Word, your stomach, or digestive system, is much less likely to cause you problems.

Treasure God's Word. Keep God first place in your life. The kingdom of God is what He tells you to seek first. When you do this, you will treasure the Words of God. You will treasure your Bible.

Thank you, Lord, for giving us the written Word.

> Job 23:12 - I have not departed from the commandment of His lips; I have treasured the Words of His mouth more than my necessary food.

# July 26

Do you have a child, or adult, with mental problems of any kind? Was someone born with a problem? Autism is one example. Learning difficulties is another example. Is someone you know suffering with Alzheimer's, dementia or other mental problems?

The scripture below is excellent for praying over anyone with any of these problems. You want them to have a sound mind. One person has made great progress with people in several of these categories by having them meditate on scriptures. This is one you could use.

God heals. It doesn't have to be the flu, a broken leg, or any common thing. God heals. He wants everyone healed. I know people who have given up because the healing was not done quickly. Don't quit. God heals.

Mental problems are just as real as a broken leg. Birth defects can be healed. I knew a man whose daughter had to have part of the brain removed. They worked with people who believed in healing, and his daughter has made great progress.

Nothing is too difficult for God, and there is nothing He won't address. Trust God. Seek God for help. Let Him show you how to pray, what to do.

> 2 Timothy 1:7 - For God has not given us a spirit of fear, but of power and of love and of a sound mind.

## July 27

The human body was made to function in certain ways. Many things are natural and normal. Elimination of waste is something that is normal. There are many areas in the body that do this, but normally we think of the kidneys and bowels.

When the body does not function properly, that is a health issue. The words of your mouth are powerful. Using the scripture below can remind your body how it is supposed to function.

This also gets a picture in your mind of the proper function of the body. True, when you do not eat properly, that can cause problems. Also, dehydration can cause problems.

Seek God to see if you have caused the problem, and what the solution is. Seek natural information to obtain more knowledge. Work on your mind and your body with scripture.

> Mark 7:18–19
> 18 So He said to them, "Are you thus without understanding also? Do you not perceive that whatever enters a man from outside cannot defile him,
> 19 because it does not enter his heart but his stomach, and is eliminated, thus purifying all foods?"

## July 28

Have you ever suffered a burn? Almost every one has. You accidentally touch the rack in the oven is all it takes. There is a burn. Some burns are minor and heal very quickly. Some ice on your finger after you touched the rack, and it can be fine very shortly.

When someone is badly burned, it can take the body a long time to recover. Many burn victims need to be in the hospital for a long time. Then, they often need surgery, possibly plastic surgery.

Three Hebrew men were thrown in a raging fire, and came out without even the smell of smoke on them. God is no respecter of people. They believed for it, and God met their expectations.

If you, or someone you know, is burned, start prayer as soon as possible. Believe God for a miracle with their healing. Pray for the people attending them to be given wisdom to meet their needs.

> Daniel 3:27 - And the satraps, administrators, governors, and the king's counselors gathered together, and they saw these men on whose bodies the fire had no power; the hair of their head was not singed nor were their garments affected, and the smell of fire was not on them.

## July 29

Have you found yourself in a position where you do not have food or water? That is not God. He does not ever want you without food or water. There are many people who are suffering from dehydration, doctors tell them that, but they are simply not drinking enough water.

If you know people without food or water, give them what you can. Help them find supplies. If you are not drinking enough water, but it is available, that is your fault. Your body needs water.

The scripture below tells you that God wants you having food and water. When people have no money and no food, do what you can to help them. That is not the time to give them a scripture, that is a time to give food.

After necessities have been met, then you can start teaching people that when they learn to trust God, He will help them. That is the time to start sharing scriptures and teaching people about God.

> Isaiah 49:10 - They shall neither hunger nor thirst, neither heat nor sun shall strike them; for He who has mercy on them will lead them, even by the springs of water He will guide them.

## July 30

When a woman is pregnant, there are women who spend much time in painful labor. That is not necessary. God does not require that of his children. Pharaoh wanted the male Hebrew children to be killed by the midwives. The scripture below is their answer.

God protected the Hebrew children when they were in Egypt. Certainly, He would do the same for born-again women. If you are pregnant, using the verse below to speed up your labor time would be beneficial.

If you would use this scripture in regular meditation before and during a pregnancy, it will get this implanted into your mind, your body, and your spirit. Everything will work together for an easy birth.

One family I have heard of had several children. Then they learned what God will do if you have a baby by faith. They set the day for the birth, went to the hospital each time, and the baby was born quickly and with no problems. They had at least four more children as a result of this.

> Exodus 1:19 - And the midwives said to Pharaoh, "Because the Hebrew women are not like the Egyptian women; for they are lively and give birth before the midwives come to them."

# July 31

The verse below is about the righteous man, those who trust in God. Today, that is a born-again Christian. God will protect you, He will guard you. What many people do not realize is that this is not automatic.

You have to trust God. As a reminder, God has an enemy here on earth. The devil does not want you to know that you have a right to no broken bones. He doesn't want you to know anything that is in the Bible.

A broken bone would be under the curse of the law. It would be included in Deuteronomy 28:61. You know that you are redeemed from the curse of the law. (Galatians 3:13) These are all good scriptures to meditate on. You don't want a broken leg as a child, a broken hip when you are old.

Learn to walk in divine health. Learn to walk free from the curse of the law. Find scriptures that minister to you, and read them out loud every day. This is called meditating the Word.

Some people change their scriptures often, some use the same ones for years. The important thing is that you use a scripture till you have it built into your mind and your spirit. They are all health to you.

> Psalm 34:20 - He guards all his bones; not one of them is broken.

## August 1

Your health encompasses every part of your body. The scripture below could be used for many problems. It could be used for someone with hearing problems, that your ear would be one that hears as the learned.

Many people have a problem speaking. A child with autism often has problems in how they speak, or they do not speak at all. There are learning disorders where the child often has problems speaking.

This verse does not have to be used with health issues, it is good for every day purposes, to improve your speaking, and to improve your hearing. God is interested in every part of your life.

God wants you healthy, He wants you understanding His teachings. This is a verse to use for every bit of that.

> Isaiah 50:4 - "The Lord GOD has given me the tongue of the learned, that I should know how to speak a word in season to him who is weary. He awakens me morning by morning, He awakens my ear to hear as the learned.

# August 2

Do you have problems with your flesh, or your overall health? What you eat has a lot to do with this. You don't have to become a fanatic over your eating. You don't have to be at the point that no one wants to socialize with you.

In Daniel, it is told, that Daniel and three others from Israel with him, chose not to eat the king's delicacies. Many people say that they only ate vegetables. This is called a Daniel fast. Scriptures say that Daniel purposed not to eat the king's meat or drink his wine. Many meats are not kosher.

Daniel and the three got permission to do this as a test for ten days. After just ten days, they looked much better than the others who ate the king's meat and drank his wine. So, they were allowed to continue.

Check your food. Are you eating things just because they are popular, or are you looking for things that most dietitians think are healthy? I say most, this is an area where there seems to be no agreement!

Pray, ask God what you should do. He will lead you. See for yourself what ten days of eating some good things, or refusing some things, does for you. God will lead you.

> Daniel 1:15 - And at the end of ten days their features appeared better and fatter in flesh than all the young men who ate the portion of the king's delicacies.

## August 3

Do you come from a family where thinning hair is normal with old age, even bald heads for men? Did you know that you can use scripture to stop this from happening? People have used this, and similar scriptures, to stop this balding.

Paul was on a ship, they thought the ship was going to go down because of a storm. Paul promised them that God would protect them. Not a single hair will fall. I do know of people who have used this and other scriptures very successfully.

The scriptures are medicine, they are true. Not just in the area of healing. For healing scriptures are actually medicine. They help you to maintain your health. Many Christians have no concept of what scripture will do for you.

You can be healed, you can be prosperous, you can learn to draw peace, joy, and other fruits to you, in the midst of a storm. Grief, unforgiveness, emotions in this range will rob you of what God has for you. With the use of scripture, all of these can be overcome.

Learn to set your faith, even for your hair, and watch God fulfill His promises to you. God responds to faith. Without faith you cannot please God. (Hebrews 11:6)

> Acts 27:34 - Therefore I urge you to take nourishment, for this is for your survival, since not a hair will fall from the head of any of you."

## August 4

Jesus and the disciples passed a blind man. The disciples asked about why he was blind. Jesus made it clear it was not because of sin that the man was blind, but He was going to heal the man that he might know God.

The Message Bible says there was no cause-effect involved in the man being blind. Don't look at who you can blame if a baby has medical problems. Today, we are learning more and more about birth defects. If science has a cure, that is great.

God always has a cure. He wants people well. He wants people healthy and whole. Learn to look to God. He may direct you to a doctor, He may do an instant cure. Learn to look to God. Learn to follow where you are led.

The Bible is true. God never changes. Choose to believe God. Choose to believe the Bible.

> John 9:6–7
> 6 When He had said these things, He spat on the ground and made clay with the saliva; and He anointed the eyes of the blind man with the clay.
> 7 And He said to him, "Go, wash in the pool of Siloam" (which is translated, Sent). So he went and washed, and came back seeing.

## August 5

Have you fallen? This could be a spiritual fall in the verse below, but for now, look at people who have physically fallen. Possibly something was broken, possibly bruises, some damage to the body. God wants those healed. All sickness and disease are under the curse.

Do you know someone who is bowed over? This can be a bone problem, or could be caused by severe arthritis. God wants all sickness and all diseases healed. His Son, Jesus, paid the price for all of these problems at the cross.

There are so many things which people think they have to put up with. You have a right to be free from all sickness and from all disease. The first thing you have to do is to be convinced. You have to find this truth in the Bible.

Then, you have to renew your mind to these truths. The verse below gives you a visual of being healed. Using this verse to meditate can be a help for some people. Combining this with other verses can be helpful.

Another thing that is available is taking authority over sickness. Learning that God has given you tools to use is good. Then, seeking the Holy Spirit to find which tool is best each time is something you can develop as you grow.

> Psalm 145:14 - The LORD upholds all who fall, and raises up all who are bowed down.

## August 6

Why is there sickness and disease in the world? Didn't God create the world perfect? Why does it seem that sicknesses are getting worse? There are so many more than there used to be. What is all the cause of this?

The answer to this is with man, not with God. God created the world perfect. He created man perfect, but He left man in charge of the earth. He only gave man one rule, just one. And man could not keep it. Man was not to eat of the tree of good and evil.

God formed Eve from man. Man originally had all parts in him, but God took the female parts and put them in Eve. Satan came to Eve and told her to eat. She saw it was good. She ate. She offered it to Adam. Adam could have said, "No." He didn't. This handed the keys to earth to Satan. Not forever, but for the terms of the lease.

This allowed Satan to do things he had been blocked from. God sent Jesus to the world. He brought the light, those who choose to live the way He taught, may walk free of sickness. They may walk in divine health. Men loved the darkness, if they choose to walk in the darkness, their deeds are evil.

> John 3:19 - And this is the con-
> demnation, that the light has come
> into the world, and men loved
> darkness rather than light, because
> their deeds were evil.

219

## August 7

Peace is essential to good health. When you are not at peace, your mind is disturbed. Your mental health is at risk. This can cause problems in your body. This can cause problems with your heart.

Learn to walk in peace. When things around you are going bad, how can you do this? The only way you can do this is to give your cares to Jesus. You can't handle them, He can.

It may not be easy to learn how to do this. But for your health, it is essential to learn how to do it. What if you caused the problem that you are having? You have to forgive yourself.

One example is, you bought a new car, you bought new furniture, then your job had a problem and now you can't pay for everything! Start by forgiving yourself. Seek God for help, what do you need to do?

Worry won't help. It can make things worse. A heart attack would be worse. Lean on God. He has answers to help you out of your problems. Learn to walk in peace at all times. If God tells you to sell the car, do it. Receive peace.

> John 14:27 - Peace I leave with you, My peace I give to you; not as the world gives do I give to you. Let not your heart be troubled, neither let it be afraid.

## August 8

The words of your mouth are very important. They affect your health. If you keep speaking sickness, you will have sickness. If you speak good health, expect good health.

If you have someone in agreement with you for your health, that magnifies your faith. God has given you a measure of faith. It is your job to exercise your faith, to watch it grow.

The world does not understand the importance of this. However, doctors do know that your attitude can help. They have witnessed miracles, but not all of medical science understand the importance of trusting God.

Most doctors know that your attitude plays a strong role in your health. They have watched people that they thought would never live, recover and be fine. Those healings cannot be explained medically.

The Christian has the Word to tell them God wants you well. He has provided healing for you through His Word. Study the Word, learn to exercise your faith. Be a doer of the Word.

> 2 Corinthians 4:13 - And since we have the same spirit of faith, according to what is written, "I believed and therefore I spoke," we also believe and therefore speak,

## August 9

When you are believing for a healing, you want to find several scriptures. These scriptures should contain two types of information, if possible. You should meditate scriptures that renews your mind to the fact that God wants you healed.

Another thing that helps is for you to picture yourself healed. If you are believing for a car, TV, computer, or other physical thing, seeing a picture of what you are believing for is very good.

In the same way, if there are scriptures that say what you are believing for, it is good to use those scriptures. The scripture below is good for hips, stomach muscles, strength in the abdominal area. It builds a picture in your mind.

What do you do with these scriptures? Write them down. Post a copy on your refrigerator, your bathroom mirror, other places where you will see them. Put them with your Bible. Scriptures are medicine. Read them out loud several times a day.

> Job 40:16 - See now, his strength is in his hips, and his power is in his stomach muscles.

## August 10

What is the best way to pray? Use scriptures. Scriptures are healing, not only to your body, but to your emotions. They can also be healing to a car, or relationships.

For healing, find scriptures telling you that God heals. Then, also find scriptures telling you what you want to happen. Sometimes this is harder, but just think, they are there. For instance, cancer, there are scriptures telling you that nothing is impossible to God. Use those scriptures. ( Luke1:37).

Read the scriptures you choose out loud daily. Reading scriptures is never vain repetitions. It is pleasing to God. It is meditation of God's Word. Something which He told Joshua to do. (Joshua 1:8).

I have known this for years, but had not been using scriptures daily in my prayers. I added some scriptures, and God said to me, "Thank you for using scriptures as you pray." I thought, "How simple." I knew to do that, but hadn't.

Sometimes, I wait, wanting to find 'the perfect scripture.' Ask God. He will supply those for you.

> Matthew 6:7 - And when you pray, do not use vain repetitions as the heathen do. For they think that they will be heard for their many words

By Patricia L. Whipp

## August 11

Your eating has a lot to do with your health. If you eat a piece of candy, it is not a sin. It probably will not hurt your health. But if you eat only candy, your health will definitely be badly affected.

One woman I knew had a mother who started eating a popular snack cake. That is all she ate for several years. Her health had to be affected. Her daughter was born again. She had others start praying for her mother, and they broke that. The woman regained her senses.

Peter was given a vision. In that vision, all sorts of things which had been forbidden to eat were on a sheet, and Peter was told, "Take and eat." He was horrified, but God was showing him they were OK. The Kosher laws were released to Peter. Gentiles were allowed into Christianity.

Today, we have all sorts of food ideas. Learn what works for your body, what is healthy for you. Learn to be sensible, not to be legalistic. Do not judge others over their food habits. Learn to be tolerant.

> 1 Corinthians 10:23 - All things are lawful for me, but not all things are helpful; all things are lawful for me, but not all things edify.

## August 12

The disciples were concerned because there was a child who would fall into a fire, or into water, and they could not cast the demon out of the child. The father then took the child to Jesus. He immediately delivered the child.

When the disciples asked Jesus why they had not been successful, His answer is in the scripture below. Note: the disciples did not give up. They continued, learned, and succeeded later in the Bible.

What do you learn from this? First, don't give up. Exercise your faith, build it, and continue. Secondly, nothing will be impossible to you. Whether you are believing for a healing for yourself, or someone else, nothing will be impossible to you.

> Matthew 17:20 - So Jesus said to them, "Because of your unbelief; for assuredly, I say to you, if you have faith as a mustard seed, you will say to this mountain, 'Move from here to there,' and it will move; and nothing will be impossible for you.

## August 13

God created ears and eyes when He created the universe. Animals, birds, fish, man all have eyes and ears. There are times when these do not function correctly.

God has helped man to do many things to improve both vision and hearing. Glasses today aid with vision, surgery is done on the eyes today that was not even thought of 20 years ago.

The same is true with the ears. There are hearing aids that are more complex, and enhance hearing far greater, than there were 20 years ago.

God will heal eyes and ears. He also aids doctors and has aided the medical field in this area, as is happening in many areas. If you have problems with vision or hearing, seek God. Find out what He wants you to do.

No matter how or where you obtain your healing, use scriptures. If you go to a doctor, scriptures are medicine, and they will enhance what the doctor does.

The scripture below helps you to renew your mind, as well as your body, for both your eyes and your ears.

Matthew 13:16 - But blessed are your eyes for they see, and your ears for they hear;

## August 14

Some children are born with learning disabilities. Some people develop them for different reasons. Some people develop mental problems as they get older.

One doctor has done medical studies on many of these people. This doctor has found that many people can be greatly helped by meditating the Word of God.

This makes sense. Scripture tells us the Word is medicine to the flesh. (Proverbs 4:22) So, the fact that scriptures help with mental abilities makes sense.

I would suggest following the same pattern for learning disabilities that you follow for any other illness. Find general healing scriptures, and scriptures which describe what you want as the end result.

With the scripture below, you build wisdom, righteousness, sanctification and redemption into their mind. Those all sound like good qualities to have.

Pray, and trust God to bring what is needed to the person being prayed for.

> 1 Corinthians 1:30 - But of Him you are in Christ Jesus, who became for us wisdom from God—and righteousness and sanctification and redemption—

## August 15

A very important lesson to learn is to walk in peace. When you are in fear, anxiety, stress, or other negative attitudes, you are not at peace. When that happens, your heart is not good, your blood pressure often becomes high.

Jesus gave you His peace. It is in you. When you get stressed, call peace to rise up. If you are in unforgiveness, you need to deal with that to be able to walk in peace. If you are judging others, you need to deal with that to be able to walk in peace.

Learning to walk in peace is a lifetime lesson. You will think you have achieved it, and suddenly things will come up to steal your peace. The devil is a thief, he is just as happy stealing your peace as he is stealing goods from you.

When you realize you are not in peace, stop, find out why! What is stealing your peace? What can you do about it? Then, take the steps you need to take to get your peace back.

> Isaiah 54:10 - For the mountains shall depart and the hills be removed, but My kindness shall not depart from you, nor shall My covenant of peace be removed," says the LORD, who has mercy on you.

## August 16

God wants you well. He wants you to be healthy. This is how man was created, and God never changes. What He wanted for Adam, He wants for you.

If you have this well-established in your mind, it is easier to achieve what God wants for you. Don't have any doubts. Don't ever think that God wants you sick for a season. You may learn things during an illness, but that was because God had your attention, not because that was what He wanted.

Often, when accidents happen or illnesses come, people loose sight of the primary purpose of their being here. You are to seek first the Kingdom of God. You are to witness to others about the goodness of God.

God is good. The devil is evil. Don't ever forget that. Sickness is not good. God does not use evil, He did not create evil.

When the day comes that you move on to heaven, you want to be able to say the same thing that Paul said in the verse below. Keep this as your goal. You may have set backs, but make fighting the good fight of faith your goal.

> 2 Timothy 4:7 - I have fought the good fight, I have finished the race, I have kept the faith.

## August 17

The bones are what shapes the body. They are the strength of the body. If the bones are brittle, not in good shape, it puts your whole body at risk.

Medical science is doing much in this area, but doctors disagree on what is healthy, and what is good.

What can you do to protect your bones? Read the Word of God. Pray the Word of God. Speak the Word of God. The scripture below says, "It will be strength to your bones."

What is "It"? This is referring to God's teachings, which is the Word of God, which is the Bible. So, as you are meditating on scriptures, you are strengthening your bones.

Also, speak the pure, the good, give praise reports often. Get in the habit each day of looking at what God has done for you that day. Thank Him for what He has done for you. Your good reports make your bones healthy.

> Proverbs 3:8 - It will be health to your flesh, and strength to your bones.

## August 18

A fever is part of many illnesses, but it is something that you can always speak to. Getting the fever down will help with the total healing. You do not want someone continuing with a fever.

As you pray for sicknesses, fevers are often included. However, the scriptures below give you proof that you can command the fever to leave. Jesus touched Peter's mother-in-law and her fever left immediately.

Learn to speak to things like fever, blisters, pain, and watch these go. Another very important thing is to learn to listen to your spirit. God knows best what is needed at any given time. Let God lead you in what you pray for.

God wants you totally well, feeling good, walking with joy, and peace in your heart. He wants you strong and doing good. Learn to walk as He guides you into this.

> Matthew 8:14–15
> 14 Now when Jesus had come into Peter's house, He saw his wife's mother lying sick with a fever.
> 15 So He touched her hand, and the fever left her. And she arose and served them.

## August 19

Cares, anxieties, stress, these are all bad for your health. God tells you this over and over. Doctors tell you this, over and over. When the Bible and the doctors agree, then it must really be bad for you.

If you aren't sick, these can make you sick. If you are sick, these will only make your disease worse. Learn to walk in peace. Jesus gave you His peace. Peace is healthy, and will help you. Draw on the peace of Jesus.

Have the doctors told you there is no hope? They don't know your Jesus. He is your hope. He is your deliverer, He is your healer. Jesus doesn't know 'no hope.' He is your hope. Jesus died for your healing.

Any cares that you have, cast them on Jesus. He knows what to do with them. You do not. Trust God, and walk healed.

1 Peter 5:7 - casting all your care upon Him, for He cares for you.

## August 20

Do you have problems with your stomach or your digestive system? Watch the words of your mouth. Fill your mouth with God's Word. God's Word is medicine to you. Your digestive system should function better when you are speaking God's Word.

The words of your mouth are very important. I recently heard of a way you can prove this. Make some rice, at least three cups. Get three new containers. Write on the containers. Mark one, "Good words," one "Ignore," and the other "Bad words." Then, for a week, speak good words to the one marked "Good words" and speak bad to the one marked "Bad words."

Good words are, "You are good, you are great, I love you" etc. I would read some scriptures. Bad words are not cussing, they are, "You are horrible, you are no good, you will never be worthwhile."

The person who did this brought a picture. The one marked "Good words" had one piece of mold; the one marked "Ignored" had several pieces of mold; the one marked "Bad words" was filled with mold. It was very impressive.

The same thing happens to your body, when you speak good over it, it thrives. When you speak bad over it, you cause problems. Train yourself to speak positive words.

> Proverbs 18:20 - A man's stomach shall be satisfied from the fruit of his mouth; from the produce of his lips he shall be filled.

By Patricia L. Whipp

## August 21

Do you have a problem the doctors do not know what to do about, or no one knows what is going on? God knows! As you learn to seek God, He will either heal you, or get you to the right person who does know what to do.

God does not always do things the same way, He uses a variety of methods. Some people He heals immediately, some people He sends to specialists. Jesus put clay on one man's eyes and told him to go wash it off.

Some people only want to receive certain ways. That does not line up with the Word. For years, I quoted a scripture which I thought meant I would never have to have cataract surgery. What did God do? Told me to go have surgery.

Don't try to tell God how to do things. BUT, do realize that, when doctors don't know, when people don't know, God knows how to get something done. You find scriptures for what you want, meditate those scriptures. That is part of what you need to do.

Listen to God, that is another thing you need to do. When He tells you to speak, to go, follow His directions, and watch miracles happen.

Luke 1:37 - For with God nothing will be impossible.

August 22

The following scripture is for a day when wisdom returns. This certainly is a season in the Christian life when more Christians are walking in wisdom. Many people are returning to basics and to the filling of the Holy Spirit.

When Jesus was on the earth, the deaf had their hearing restored and the blind had their sight restored. We should start seeing this in the days ahead. Anyone can minister to people, even in the areas that many people consider difficult.

Don't hesitate to pray for healing for people. Get enough Word into you that you are not afraid to pray for someone to receive their sight. Are you thinking, "What if they don't receive it?" I ask, "What if they do?"

If someone doesn't manifest a healing immediately, you have sown a seed. Tell them that God heals, God wants them healed, and to keep believing for the manifestation. Do not ignore praying for people because you walk in doubt. Get rid of your doubt.

God wants His people healed. God wants non-Christians healed as a sign and a wonder. It draws people to Jesus.

> Isaiah 29:18 - In that day the deaf shall hear the words of the book, and the eyes of the blind shall see out of obscurity and out of darkness.

## August 23

Many people think that Paul had a sickness. Some even believe that it was from God. If you think either of these, go to the Bible and read the verse.

Paul was being attacked by a messenger from Satan. A demon was attacking Paul. Paul sought God three times to get rid of it. Three times God told him that His (God's) grace was sufficient.

When Jesus died on the cross, we were given authority over all the power of the enemy. We have authority over the attacks of the enemy. We need to learn to exercise this authority.

This is the same thing that Paul had to do when he went to God about the thorn in his flesh. God told him three times what he needed to do. Apparently, he heard (understood) what God said after the third time. He must have exercised his authority.

You can do the same thing when you are sick. Paul was not sick, but you have authority over sickness. Learn to exercise your authority over sickness.

> 2 Corinthians 12:9 - And He said to me, "My grace is sufficient for you, for My strength is made perfect in weakness." Therefore most gladly I will rather boast in my infirmities, that the power of Christ may rest upon me.

## August 24

God is the Father of mercies and of all comfort. As we are healed, it is nice to have mercy and comfort. God has compassion. He understands more than we realize.

It has taken me a long time to learn that God understands. His first-begotten Son lived as a man on this earth. He suffered all things. He never sinned, that is why He had to learn obedience. Because He had never been disobedient, He had to learn about obedience.

God has far more understanding of what is happening to us than we realize. He understands our desire for health. He understands our desire for things. He also has provided all things for us.

When sickness tries to come on you, seek God. Find your healing in the scriptures. For many things you can simply take authority. He has given you authority over the enemy.

Learn to immediately seek good health when symptoms first start. Don't wait to see if you are going to get sick.

Praise God, thank Him for His mercies and blessings that He bestows on you and those you pray for.

> 2 Corinthians 1:3 - Blessed be the God and Father of our Lord Jesus Christ, the Father of mercies and God of all comfort,

By Patricia L. Whipp

## August 25

Have you heard of the maimed being made whole? It is in the Bible. As Jesus prayed for people, it often happened immediately.

When He prayed for the multitudes, miracles happened, very unusual miracles in the minds of many people.

These things are happening today. Not as many are seen in America as elsewhere, but they are happening and, if we will continue praying for the sick, we will see more and more of these.

Are you believing for a total miracle? Don't quit. Hold fast to your faith. Don't doubt. God has miracles available, and why not you?

When people see miracles, they are more open to receive Jesus. Pray for revival around the world. Pray for people to receive Jesus.

Pray for healing revivals. Pray for healing revivals around the world. Pray for healing revivals in America.

> Matthew 15:31 - So the multitude marveled when they saw the mute speaking, the maimed made whole, the lame walking, and the blind seeing; and they glorified the God of Israel.

## August 26

Do you have problems walking? Do you stumble or fall easily? That is a part of your health. That is something that Jesus paid the price for you to be free from. If you are not believing for freedom from these problems, start believing now.

There can be many problems which cause something of this nature. It can be a deformity of the foot, leg, hip, or can be caused by problems with balance. That can come from a problem in the brain, or the thyroid, or other structural deformities.

Is there a missing foot? God has spare parts in heaven, and it is time to start believing for these creative miracles. God has no shortage on what He wants to do. He can visualize things we haven't even considered.

Part of why it takes us time to receive these healings is imagining the possibilities. God wants you well, and no price is too great. The price does not have to be money, the price can be your believing.

Trust God and let Him show you. Pray and believe.

> Proverbs 3:23 - Then you will walk safely in your way, and your foot will not stumble.

By Patricia L. Whipp

## August 27

Some people think that God will not heal everything, for example bones. They have said that for bones you have to go to a doctor. God is interested and wants every part of your body healthy.

Today there are all sorts of ads for white teeth. All tooth paste seems to contain a whitener for your teeth. That is a major concern with beauty consultants. I have seen dentists who have ads stating, "We whiten teeth."

On his death bed, Jacob prophesied to his twelve sons. To Judah, in part Jacob said, "His teeth shall be whiter than milk." You can use that as a picture of your teeth being white, and if they are white, that there is no cavity in them.

There is no part of your body that God does not want well, healthy, and functioning as it should be. Trust God, believe Him, and be healthy.

> Genesis 49:12 - His eyes are darker than wine, and his teeth whiter than milk.

# August 28

Jesus went back to where He had turned the water into wine. There, a nobleman came and asked Jesus to please come and pray for his son. Jesus told him to return home and said that his son would live.

When the nobleman had returned home, he checked with the servants to see when his son started getting better. His son started getting better at the same hour that he had talked to Jesus.

In this case, the son had a fever, and the indication is that the fever left at the time Jesus talked to the nobleman. Trust God, He wants you well more than you do. Do you have a fever? God will heal that, and whatever is causing the fever.

There is no sickness or disease that God cannot heal. He wants you well. Trust Him. These things happened before Jesus went to the cross. God has always wanted His people well. Now that Jesus suffered all illness for you, how much more you have as evidence of God's desire to have you healthy.

> John 4:52 - Then he inquired of them the hour when he got better. And they said to him, "Yesterday at the seventh hour the fever left him."

## August 29

Jesus sent His twelve disciples out to preach the kingdom of God and to heal the sick. They were amazed at what they could do. Have you talked to others about the kingdom of God? Have you prayed for the sick?

These are simple steps, they are also steps which Jesus told all believers to do. If you have started doing this, continue. If you haven't started, start today. Do you take a bus to work? Tell the person beside you about Jesus.

In a restaurant, it's not easy to talk to people at other tables, but I find the servers are always available to tell them about things. Normally, I have a book with me to read, and often I will get asked about my book. Great witnessing tool.

Pray for others, on the street, at work, at home. I had a minister when I first started with the Word of Faith teachings say, "If you can't do these things at home, you can't do them anywhere." It turned out to be excellent advice. Don't be pushy, just informative.

Pray for the sick, at work, at home, next door.

Luke 9:2 - He sent them to preach the kingdom of God and to heal the sick.

## August 30

God wants you healthy, He wants you well. There are many methods in the Bible that have been used for healing. There is no statement that says it must be done one way. The scripture below is from when the 12 disciples were sent out two by two.

Note: in this verse it says that they anointed with oil many who were sick. We also find elsewhere that you can anoint people with oil for healing. This does not mean you do it every time. But it is a way that is scriptural and is used in the Bible.

We have previously talked about just praying, meditating scriptures, taking authority over the thief.

There are many ways for people to be healed. Do not think that you have to anoint everyone with oil. Do not think you will not get healed if someone did not anoint you with oil. However, do not discard this method. It is good, it works, and many are healed this way.

> Mark 6:13 - And they cast out many demons, and anointed with oil many who were sick, and healed them.

## August 31

Do you have problems with your flesh or your skin? God is as interested in your flesh and your skin being healthy as He is about any part of you. Is your skin discolored? I believe that is something God will help you with as well.

God loves you. He loves you as much as He loves Jesus. Learn to trust God, and to believe that He wants you well. The primary thing is believe. Just because thoughts that He won't heal this come to you does not mean that you don't believe. When those thoughts come, tell them to leave you in the name of Jesus.

The scripture below is one you can use to help you visualize the skin or flesh being renewed. True, this was spoken to dry bones, but how much more can God replace skin and flesh on living bones! No healing is impossible for God.

Having other people pray for you, or agree with you in prayer, is always a good idea. Trust God, believe, and when necessary, be patient.

> Ezekiel 37:6 - I will put sinews on you and bring flesh upon you, cover you with skin and put breath in you; and you shall live. Then you shall know that I am the LORD.

# September 1

How do you fight the good fight of faith? You do it by being a doer of the Word. How do you be a doer of the Word? (James 1:22) What does that mean? That means you study the Word, you learn what God expects you to do.

The first step is to seek first the kingdom of God. (Matthew 6:33) That is a decision. Tell God that you want to be a doer, you want to seek the Kingdom. That simple. Then some steps for you to follow, actions that you can take are to meditate the Word. (Joshua 1:8) Find a scripture that you want to study, read it out loud several times a day.

Read the Bible, study the Bible. Learn what it says. God says that His people are destroyed for a lack of knowledge. (Hosea 4:6) A lack of knowledge of what? A lack of knowledge of what the Bible says.

You cannot go to church once a week, listen to a sermon, not learn anything, and fight the good fight of faith. You need to find a church that teaches the Bible, the truth. You need to take notes, be a learner, be a student of the Word. Then you can use what you have learned to fight the good fight of faith.

> 1 Timothy 6:12 - Fight the good fight of faith, lay hold on eternal life, to which you were also called and have confessed the good confession in the presence of many witnesses.

245

By Patricia L. Whipp

## September 2

Learning to live in peace is very important to your health. Your body does not handle stress well. It is designed for peace, not stress. This world operates in stress.

The scriptures below tell you a way to maintain peace, and to strive for peace in the world. See the world at peace. Pray for peace. As you pray, if you will believe your prayers, then you see peace coming. You believe that peace is here.

This sounds unbelievable to some, but has actually been studied scientifically. The part of the brain which is active changes when you pray in tongues.

I believe you will find people who pray in tongues are energized. Scripture says that it is like charging a battery. (Jude 20)

Pray using scriptures and pray in tongues. Pray for the world, that we may lead a quiet and peaceable life.

> 1 Timothy 2:1–2
> 1 Therefore I exhort first of all that supplications, prayers, inter-cessions, and giving of thanks be made for all men,
> 2 for kings and all who are in authority, that we may lead a quiet and peaceable life in all godliness and reverence.

## September 3

What are you saying? When you don't feel well, does everyone know it? Has the doctor told you that you have a disease, maybe the worst case he has ever seen? Does everyone know the doctor's report?

Or, have you had prayer for the problems you have? Have you received your healing? Are you talking the healing? Does no one know the doctor's report?

Which of the above situations are most likely going to have a positive outcome? Which one will lead to an active life? Which one will lead to divine health?

Your tongue can cause you lots of problems or lots of blessings. God created the earth by speaking. If God is your Father, then you are supposed to imitate Him. You are to speak to things and watch them happen. That includes speaking to your body.

This includes your thoughts. Out of the heart the mouth speaks. (Luke 6:45) If you think you are sick, if you dwell on it, you will bring that to pass. I know of two people who died because they held on to negative doctors' reports.

Watch your tongue, and keep your thoughts in line with the Word of God.

> Proverbs 18:21 - Death and life are in the power of the tongue, and those who love it will eat its fruit.

## September 4

You are told to raise the dead! Actually, that is not new, people have been raised from the dead in both the Old and the New Testaments. A few of these follow:

Elijah raised a son of a widow that he lodged with. (1 Kings 17:19-22) Elisha raised the son of a couple that had provided a room for him. (2 Kings 4:32-35)

Jesus raised several people from the dead. There were two children, as well as Lazarus. (John 11:38-44)

Peter raised a woman named Tabitha from the dead. (Acts 9:40)

Paul raised a man who fell out of a window from the dead. (Acts 20:9)

We have many ministries in the last few centuries that have recorded instances of people being raised from the dead. Some people think that things like leprosy or cancer cannot be healed. Anything which is established in the Bible is available for a believer to do.

Find your scriptures and act on those.

Matthew 10:8 - Heal the sick, cleanse the lepers, raise the dead, cast out demons. Freely you have received, freely give.

## September 5

Are you having problems walking? This could be caused by many things. There could be problems with your feet, knees, legs, hips, or just your toes. It could also be balance problems which may be part of the thyroid.

No matter what the cause is, God wants it healed. He wants every single part of you whole and well. Learn to trust God for your total health. Believe Him, find scriptures that tell you what you want healed is healed.

What you need to do is build a vision in you. You need to see yourself walking completely normal. This is why you need scriptures talking about walking normally. Without a vision, without picturing this, you can not pray for it.

Many people do not realize the importance of seeing what you are praying for. You need to picture it happening. If you can see it, and it is good, it is something in God's will, you can have it. If it is bad, you may have it, but that was not God.

God wants you well. He wants you whole. He wants the best for you.

> Zechariah 10:12 - "So I will strengthen them in the LORD, and they shall walk up and down in His name," says the LORD.

## September 6

God wants His people totally well. He wants your health completely restored. He wants your wounds totally healed. The Jews were an outcast, health and restoration is what He wanted for the Jews.

Christians are an outcast in some areas of the world. Christians are the seed of Abraham. They are grafted in. God wants no less for the Christians than He wants for the Jews. God does not change.

It is our job to accept what God wants for us, to learn how to receive, to learn what He expects of us. Things, healings, are not just zapped on someone. At times, it appears that way, but on a regular basis that is not true.

God expects you to spend time in the Word; to learn what He has for you; to learn how to pray. He also expects you to use your faith. You are to use your faith, to grow in faith.

You should spend time in praise and worship. Spend time with God. Not just at church, but in your daily life. You can do this in your everyday life. Praise God, thank Him for His love, for His patience, for His mercy.

> Jeremiah 30:17 - For I will restore health to you and heal you of your wounds,' says the LORD, 'because they called you an outcast saying: "This is Zion; no one seeks her." '

# September 7

God knows you. He knows more about you than you will ever know. Even the hairs on your head, they are all numbered. God is your healer, He is the one who can fix anything in, or on, your body.

If you come from a family where balding, or thin hair, is normal with old age, start claiming the original count of your hair to be on your head. If you build your faith in that area, it is yours.

No matter what sickness, no matter what health issue you may have, God is bigger. If you want to walk in divine health, God is available to assist you with that. Find the scriptures you want to use, and meditate on them.

Never forget the importance of the Bible. It has been given to you. It is gift to you from your heavenly Father. Yes, it is a history book, but that is just a small part of what it is. The Bible is the living Word of God. Jesus' name is called The Word of God. (Revelation 19:13)

Walk in faith. Walk in knowledge of the Word.

> Luke 12:7 - But the very hairs of your head are all numbered. Do not fear therefore; you are of more value than many sparrows.

## September 8

You want to walk in good health. You want to be able to pray for others to be healed. You also want to be able to tell others that God heals. Healing is wonderful. It is a gift from God that you need to use and want to share.

God does expect things from His people. One of the things He wants is that you read the Bible. You learn about healing scriptures. You learn about praying. He also expects you to meditate on healing scriptures.

Meditate can sound like a strange word for a Christian. It is really quite simple. Read Bible verses out loud. Since we are talking about healing, read Bible verses that have to do with healing out loud. I recommend at least three verses. Find three that minister to you.

Meditate on these morning and night, soon you will have them memorized. It is good to review them periodically. Otherwise, you might find you left out a word, or changed a word. Reviewing a Bible verse just means looking it up.

Praise God, thank Him for His love, and for His healing.

> Psalm 1:2 - But his delight is in the law of the LORD, and in His law he meditates day and night.

## September 9

There is no one method to healing. There is no 3-step method that you use. God wants you healed and He has many plans for your healing. Meditating God's Word, setting your faith, these are all good and are all ways God heals.

The scripture below is not just used for healing, but it is very good for healing. This scripture says, "This is the confidence...," this is confidence; no 'doubt,' no 'will it work,' no 'what if.' Ask anything according to His will.

We know that healing is God's will. We have many scriptures that tell us it is. So, if we ask anything, that means healing. That means cancer go! That means deafness go! There are many scriptures about eye sight and deafness going.

Confidence. This scripture is your confidence. You do need to find the scriptures promising what you are believing for, but if God says something is yours, this scripture gives you the confidence you need to stand.

> 1 John 5:14–15
> 14 Now this is the confidence that we have in Him, that if we ask anything according to His will, He hears us.
> 15 And if we know that He hears us, whatever we ask, we know that we have the petitions that we have asked of Him.

## September 10

When you have set your faith, it is helpful to have one or more scriptures showing what you are believing. This can help you hold strong with your faith, it gives you a visual picture of you healed.

Sometimes, you will use scriptures that don't talk about healing, but they show that body part working fine. This is a good way to build the picture in your mind.

God is your protector, He is a shield for you. He lifts up your head. If you had a problem with your neck, if it hurt, wouldn't the words, "He lifts up your head," give you a mental picture of your neck being healed?

Sometimes, a picture can come from a scripture that does not mean what you're believing has occurred, but every time you say that scripture, you see a picture of what you desire.

This is what I mean by saying that you need to be creative. Some people may call this thinking out of the box. Learn to be creative, as you read scriptures, let the Holy Spirit paint pictures for you. You will find useful scriptures in places you had not thought of by doing this.

> Psalm 3:3 - But You, O LORD, are a shield for me, my glory and the One who lifts up my head.

# September 11

I have had many friends who have hurt a shoulder. This can been devastating. Some may never be able to work again. I know of several people who have had surgery on their shoulders.

God wants you healed. He wants you whole. It is not His will for your shoulder to be bad. Since God is for you, and He is the One who knows how to heal your shoulder, my suggestion is to follow God's advice.

You are told to meditate the Word. That means you quote scriptures out loud, it also means to picture yourself being healed. Find healing scriptures that minister to you. The Bible is full of healing scriptures. Some speak to your spirit better than others.

Next, a scripture of the shoulder being free is a picture of your shoulder being healed. There are several verses about the yoke being removed. I would think a hurt shoulder would be like a yoke on the shoulder. The scripture below is a picture of the days after Jesus has come. That is today.

Have someone pray for your shoulder, then several times a day, quote scriptures to paint the picture in your mind and your spirit. See yourself healed.

> Isaiah 9:4 - For You have broken the yoke of his burden and the staff of his shoulder, the rod of his oppressor, as in the day of Midian.

## September 12

Have you ever had a panic attack? Do you know people who have them? They are not fun. It is like it takes over your mind. A total feeling of fear can come on someone who has that problem. That is considered a medical condition.

Normally when I fly, I sit in a window seat. I never thought about it, I just choose to sit there. One time, on a full flight, I had to sit in an aisle seat. As I sat there, the only thing to look at was the sea of people coming down the aisle. Normally, I am looking out a window. I realized that someone who had panic attacks could easily find that overwhelming.

What can someone in that condition do? Start quoting scriptures. God is your protector. Fear is of Satan. It is not from God. You have the authority over Satan. Start quoting scriptures, and you can also take authority over the fear. God is your protector. The enemies will have to flee in seven ways!

> Deuteronomy 28:7 - "The LORD will cause your enemies who rise against you to be defeated before your face; they shall come out against you one way and flee before you seven ways.

## September 13

Are you at peace? Is your heart peaceful, quiet, at rest? That is a healthy condition for it to be in. Even doctors know that. This is another area that the Bible has told us about and medical science has proven.

Learn to live at peace. Things may be messed up around you, but you can draw from God and stay at peace. Envy, jealousy, stress are all feelings that cause problems with the body. These feelings are rottenness to the bones! Could that be cancer to the bones?

No matter what the problem, we know that these cause a stress on the body, and cause health problems. If you get upset over something that happens, and you feel stress starting to rise, learn to drop the stress. Forgive if that is needed.

We have far more control over our body than most of us realize. Learn to walk in peace. The peace of God is healthy, and brings a quiet to the mind that is strengthening. Do what is necessary to maintain that peace. If it starts to lift, stop what you were going to do. Look for what direction or steps cause the peace to stay. That is also a way to start learning to hear God.

Proverbs 14:30 - A sound heart is life to the body, but envy is rottenness to the bones.

By Patricia L. Whipp

## September 14

Are you praying for others to be healed? Most people know someone who is sick, often it is a family member. Do pray for your family, your extended family, and for friends who are sick.

Don't be pushy, but I would let people who have a long term illness know that I am praying for them. Almost always I receive a thank you for my prayers. Whether the person is a believer or not, people appreciate your prayers.

When you are praying for people who are non-believers, you are an ambassador for God. There are many Christians who are non-believers when it comes to healing, or other areas where you need to use your faith. So, even with these people, you are an ambassador telling them the Good News that Jesus suffered for their health.

Be a faithful ambassador, tell the Good News that Jesus bore the stripes for their healing. Tell the Good News that God wants them well, and that is what He has always wanted.

As you tell these things, you are bringing health to these people.

> Proverbs 13:17 - A wicked messenger falls into trouble, but a faithful ambassador brings health.

## September 15

You can often tell when a person is sick by just looking at them. Their countenance is not good. Their face looks pale, drawn, their skin may look a different color. Their eyes can look sunken in their face.

But, when you are merry, laughing, enjoying life, your look is totally different. There is healing in laughing, there is a different look about a person who is cheerful.

We use the word spirit to refer to the real you. You are a spirit. We also use the word spirit to refer to your conduct, how you are acting. "That was a great game, and you had a real team spirit."

When you are sick, your conduct is usually different. You don't appear to be energetic, you don't appear to want to do things.

If you have a sickness attacking you, laugh! Laugh at the devil for thinking that he can put something like that on you. Find a funny movie and watch it. You have the victory.

> Proverbs 15:13 - A merry heart
> makes a cheerful countenance, but
> by sorrow of the heart the spirit is
> broken.

By Patricia L. Whipp

## September 16

Often, when you are sick, you become weak. God is your strength. He promises you strength many places in the Bible. For many diseases, simply using scriptures showing the promises of strength is a great way to go.

God will raise you up off of a sick bed. Sometimes, you have to take the first step in faith, but take it. Then take the next step. Sometimes, healings are very fast. Not always.

Don't expect all healings to take place the same way every time. Look at Jesus. For one man who was blind, He made mud with His spit, wiped the mud on the man's eyes, and sent Him to a place where the water is believed to have been muddy.

Some blind people were simply spoken to. God uses many different methods. He doesn't always do everything the same.

Praise God, and thank Him for strength, for health, for His love.

Psalm 68:35 - O God, You are more awesome than Your holy places. The God of Israel is He who gives strength and power to His people. Blessed be God!

## September 17

Mental conditions, oppression and depression to name a few, are bad for your health. Those are not caused by God, they are very bad for your health. You cannot be productive when you are plagued with depression.

As with any other health problems, God wants you free. He wants you walking in joy, peace, and being merry. Those all lead to good health. A merry heart does good. It is like medicine to you.

The anointing oil is used for healing. Note: the yoke of depression, and the burden on your shoulder, will all be removed and destroyed by the anointing oil.

> Isaiah 10:27 - It shall come to pass in that day that his burden will be taken away from your shoulder, and his yoke from your neck, and the yoke will be destroyed because of the anointing oil.

## September 18

Are you believing for a child? Do you want a child and so far there has been nothing? God wants you to have children. Children are a heritage from the Lord, and they are God's desire for a husband and wife.

God designed man. He made a male and a female that we might have children. This was the design He chose to use when He created the universe. When He spoke this into being, He had the whole plan created.

As with anything else that God has promised you, set your faith for a child. True, some people don't seem to need to do that, but if you are believing for a child, this is what you do. Find scriptures promising you children.

Next, meditate on those scriptures. This is how you feed and water your faith, meditation with scriptures. Don't get in a hurry, just receive. Say out loud, "I believe, I receive a child." Then thank God for your child.

> Psalm 127:3 - Behold, children are
> a heritage from the LORD, the fruit
> of the womb is a reward.

## September 19

You are made in the image of God. God is never sick, He never has pain. Do you think He wants you sick or with pain? That does not even make sense.

Your body was created to regenerate cells as you sleep. That is why it is so important to have ample sleep. Yet many people brag about how little sleep they get each night. They are robbing their health.

Science has proven the regeneration of the body. The body goes through several cycles as you sleep. Some of these cycles are when cells are actually regenerated in the body.

Everyone gets a new set of cells about every seven years. Brain cells, nerve cells, and other body cells are all regenerated.

God wants everyone healthy. He wants everyone walking in divine health. He is health, and He wants no less for His children.

> Genesis 1:27 - So God created man in His own image; in the image of God He created him; male and female He created them.

By Patricia L. Whipp

## September 20

Have you ever considered doing a fast for your health? This does not have to be a lengthy thing. It does not have to be food! Seek God and ask what He would have you do.

In Isaiah 58, God promises healing, and gives some specific promises for people who will fast unto Him.

There are many kinds of fasting. You can fast certain foods. You can fast one meal a day. You can fast TV. Many people see the word fast and panic. Seek God, see if there is something He would like you to fast for a period of time.

Using a fast to maintain your health, or improve your health, is what Daniel and his friends did. They fasted for their spiritual health. (Daniel 1:8) They chose to fast the meats, wines, and some other things that the King ate. They did this for their health.

Fasting does not change God, but it can change your health, and can increase your faith. Consider doing this for some health problems.

> Isaiah 58:11 - The LORD will guide you continually, and satisfy your soul in drought, and strengthen your bones; you shall be like a watered garden, and like a spring of water, whose waters do not fail.

## September 21

We live in the age of the New Testament. If you are born again, walking with Jesus, you are the righteousness of Jesus. (1 Corinthians 1:30) That alone should be good news to you.

God has promises for us which we can stand on and claim. They don't just fall on you, believe and receive these promises, they are available.

If this concept is new to you, seek God. Find scriptures, find the promises that speak to you. Meditate on those scriptures several times a day. When you are ready, pray for what you want. Then, receive. Say, "I receive."

From that day forward, know, and say, "I am healed." Keeping your confession steady is very important. That is the key.

Do you want your eyes to not be dim? Moses was 120 years old and his eyes were not dim. (Deuteronomy 34:7) Believe for this. Do you want to hear the voice of the Lord? He talks to you, and will continue to do so, but you need to listen, and follow what He says to do.

Here is a scripture for you to meditate on.

Isaiah 32:3 - The eyes of those who see will not be dim, and the ears of those who hear will listen.

## September 22

Learn to praise God. This is important for your healing. You may be in pain, you may have problems that need healing. BUT—you are breathing. You can hear, you can see; if this is not true, there must be something else good. Thank God for every good thing you can think of. God inhabits the praises of His people.

God does not say "no." However, words not spoken in faith, He does not even hear. Many people think He has said "no" when actually He just didn't hear you.

Go to God in faith. Start with praise. Sing praises to God. Worship Him. Draw closer to God. Learn to walk with Him.

Watch for every sign of improvement. If you can move something that you couldn't move, praise God for that. If a pain goes away, praise God for that. Don't wait to see if it comes back, praise Him immediately.

Speak to Satan, command him to not bring that pain back.

> Psalm 22:3 - But You are holy, enthroned in the praises of Israel.

## September 23

Communion is a very good thing to do for healing. Many people have only taken communion at church, but there is no reason that you need to be at church to take communion.

At home, get out your Bible, something to drink, and a small piece of bread or a cracker. You can spend some time in praise and worship if you desire to prepare yourself.

Be sure you are not in unforgiveness. If you have anyone you know you need to forgive, do so. Has this seemed too easy? It is not a complicated process. It is a good habit to develop and do at appropriate times.

Choose one of the following scripture references and have communion.

1 Corinthians 11:23-26;

Matthew 26:26-29;

Mark 14:22-25;

Luke 22:17-20

## September 24

Are you seeking healing? What are the things you need to do? The first thing you need to do is believe that God wants you well, next you need to pray, then receive your healing, and set your faith.

How do you receive your healing when you pray, or you are prayed for? Say, "I receive." That simple. The first few healings I received were so fast, and so simple, that I was not aware of any steps.

Before I had heard any of these teachings, I went to a service where a man was praying, and sometimes he was praying for legs to grow out. I thought that was odd. I had been to a shoe store that day and they could not fit me because of foot problems.

I asked for God to show me where I could find a store that carried shoes that would fit. He said, "It is easier to fix your feet." So I went up and had my feet prayed for. I went back to the same shoe store, had my feet measured again, and they were fixed.

Some things have taken years, but the manifestation of the healing always comes. Don't quit, know that God is faithful.

> Hebrews 10:36 - For you have need of endurance, so that after you have done the will of God, you may receive the promise:

## September 25

When do you receive your healing? When you say, "I receive," consider your healing received! Normally, that occurs when someone prays for you, or you pray for yourself. At that point, receive it.

Once you have received it, what is your confession? "I am healed." You don't look at what you see, you don't go by how you feel. If you are not used to doing this, and you don't think it is right, then say something like, "In the name of Jesus, I am healed," or "I am healed by the Word of God."

Start learning to get your confession lined up with your faith. Don't listen to Satan's lies to you about doing that.

John 14:13 - And whatever you ask in My name, that I will do, that the Father may be glorified in the Son.

By Patricia L. Whipp

## September 26

Sometimes, it is best to pray for specific body parts. Praying in general, "Heal her God," often works, but being very specific can be more effective.

Many people today are having knee replacements. You often see people complaining about weak knees. Many people use a cane, or a walker, because of their knees.

God wants those knees healed. He wants strength to be in them. No matter what the cause of the feebleness, God has a healing ready!

Here are two healing scriptures for the knees. Combine these with general healing scriptures and watch the strength return to the knees.

> Isaiah 35:3 - Strengthen the weak hands, and make firm the feeble knees.

> Hebrews 12:12 - Therefore strengthen the hands which hang down, and the feeble knees,

## September 27

God is not just interested in healing your physical body, He wants you totally healed. Your mind and your soul are important, also.

Some people are born with problems in the mind. Some develop problems because of something that has happened in their life. Today, we are seeing many elderly develop problems.

God has scriptures for all of these. Once again, many general scriptures have been included which you can use for the mind and the soul.

Here are two more scriptures to use for the mind and the soul. The second one is an action for you to take, as well as a scripture for you to use.

Psalm 138:3 - In the day when I cried out, You answered me, and made me bold with strength in my soul.

Romans 12:2 - And do not be conformed to this world, but be transformed by the renewing of your mind, that you may prove what is that good and acceptable and perfect will of God.

By Patricia L. Whipp

## September 28

Something which is not mentioned much lately, but is definitely a part of our day to day warfare, is the authority of the believer. You have been given authority over all power of the enemy.

Remember in the gospels, Matthew 9:14-21 and Luke 9:37-42, there was a father who had asked the disciples for help with his son, and they could not help him. Jesus cast the demon out and the son was healed.

This is an extreme and something to remember. But even with much milder problems, you can take authority over the enemy and receive healing. I have always spoken to pain, and it leaves quickly. When I stub a toe, which I manage to do fairly often, it hurts. But not for long!

One minister I heard was not getting a healing. She had a type of malaria, and none of the medications were working. Finally, she started speaking to it in the name of Jesus. One day as she was pulling herself up to a sitting position in her hospital bed, she said one last time, "Be gone in the name of Jesus." That was the last time she spoke to it. She was healed.

> Philippians 2:10 - that at the name of Jesus every knee should bow, of those in heaven, and of those on earth, and of those under the earth,

## September 29

Peace. Learning to walk in peace is important just for life. When you are fighting for a healing, it is also very important. When you are at peace, you don't have stress, anxiety, and other bad hormones running through your body.

Jesus gave you His peace. It is in you. When you are stressed, or have anxiety, the peace does not seem to be there. What you need to do is give Jesus the problems causing you to be stressed. Just hand them to Him. He knows better than you do what to do with them. Then, if you feel a calm, but you still are not aware of the peace, just call it forth. "Peace, come forth." You can feel it rise in you.

If you are praying for others, tell them to give Jesus their problems, their cares, then call forth peace.

When I have done that, I literally feel it rise up. What is best is to just walk in that peace all the time.

You do have a choice. Stay in peace.

Psalm 29:11 - The LORD will give strength to His people; the LORD will bless His people with peace.

## September 30

God heals eyes. He wants you seeing. He wants you to see the scriptures, to see Him, to know what the scriptures mean. He is just as interested in your physical eyes as He is the eyes of your understanding.

Praying for the eyes of your understanding (Ephesians 1:18) is something that is certainly good to pray for. But having understanding when you cannot physically see is not good. It is far better to have both.

God opens blind eyes today. There are people who are blind from birth receiving eye sight. God opens deaf ears today. There are people deaf from birth receiving hearing today. These are not just things from Bible times, these are available today.

The following scriptures can be used for both; people whose eyes are blind to scripture, who do not understand, and those whose physical eyes have problems.

> Psalm 146:8 - The LORD opens the eyes of the blind; the LORD raises those who are bowed down; the LORD loves the righteous.

## October 1

Don't always expect healings to be done the same way. You may see the same results, but things done differently.

The two scriptures listed below show very similar healings done two different ways. The first one is Peter with the man at the gate called Beautiful. Peter lifted the man up, and as he was lifted, he received his healing.

The second was Paul, he spoke to the man and told him to get up. The man was healed as he got up.

It is so important to listen to the instructions, and do what was said. I have watched healing lines as a word of prophecy was said. If a minister calls out a healing and says that the "right leg..."—don't go up for a problem with your elbow or your eyes. I have watched people run up for healing of anything, no matter what was called out.

God may have mercy and heal you at that time, but if you will follow instructions, you will definitely have a better experience.

> Acts 3:7 - And he took him by the right hand and lifted him up, and immediately his feet and ankle bones received strength.

> Acts 14:10 - said with a loud voice, "Stand up straight on your feet!" And he leaped and walked.

By Patricia L. Whipp

## October 2

Do you have a learning disability? Do you know someone who does? That is not from God. True, people have different levels of intelligence. But a disability is not from God.

He did not design you with that. You need to learn to cope with it as long as you have it, but that does not mean that you don't pray and believe to be free from that disability.

The following scriptures show that God has made wisdom, knowledge, and skill available to you! Someone who does not have a learning disability, but is slow in how they learn, definitely can use these scriptures to increase their ability.

People learn at different rates. As an example, mathematics is something that many people have problems with. Part of today's problems may be the way they are taught, but still math comes easily to some people, not true for others.

> Psalm 119:99 - I have more understanding than all my teachers, for Your testimonies are my meditation.

## October 3

God brought the Jews out of Egypt and led them to the promised land. There was not one feeble person among them. Do you think that there would not have been a feeble one with them if God had not healed people? It is estimated that more than 2 million people were brought out. With that many people and to have none feeble, it seems that there had to be a miracle of God involved.

God does not change. He is still the same today as He was when He brought the Jews out of Egypt. He wants His people healed.

For a Christian, this is certainly true. God has paid the price of seeing His Son beaten and die on a cross for our healing. God wants every one of us totally healed. There is nothing He wants you to suffer or to contend with.

God does not ever make anyone sick, He never delays a healing. Sometimes healings take time, but that is because the body must go through many changes for the total healing.

> Psalm 105:37 - He also brought them out with silver and gold, and there was none feeble among His tribes.

## October 4

Are you having problems with your skin or flesh? God is interested in your skin and flesh both being healthy. The skin is the outer covering, the flesh is muscles, fat, the part that covers the bones and is under the skin.

God wants every part of your body completely healthy. Many people have minor problems with the skin, blemishes that do not look good. That is not the way God designed you, and it is not what He desires for you.

You do need to take care of your body, cleaning it, and sometimes you need to put a lotion or oil on it to lubricate it. Once again, God designed it to be perfect.

As with any other problem concerning your health, find scriptures which describe what you are believing for. Then meditate these scriptures. Scriptures are health to your flesh, they are medicine for you.

> Job 10:11 - Clothe me with skin and flesh, and knit me together with bones and sinews?

## October 5

Blood is very important to your life. Without blood you will not live. There can be many diseases in the blood. There are medical practitioners who simply read the blood. They take one drop, magnify it and can see much in the blood. They often can see things which medical doctors are not trained to see.

Most diseases, if not all, can be seen in the blood. I question that we have learned all there is to know from examining the blood. I have heard of one medical doctor who left his practice to join in research of the blood. I also know of a pharmacist who left his field and treats people as a medical practitioner by reading your blood. Both of these people feel that they can do much more to help people than they could by staying in the field they trained for.

There have been several times when I have used the following scripture over problems that the doctors were seeing in the blood. You can use these scriptures for problems which do not start in the blood, but can be seen in the blood.

There are other scriptures as well that are good. This is just one of many.

> Ezekiel 16:6 - "And when I passed by you and saw you struggling in your own blood, I said to you in your blood, 'Live!' Yes, I said to you in your blood, 'Live!'

## October 6

The health of your mind and your soul are both important to God. He wants you mentally healthy. The word strength is frequently used in scripture to refer to health. If you are weak, you are not healthy. So in the same manner, your mind and your soul both need to be strong. If they are feeble, you may not be thinking correctly.

The term to be renewed from the Greek means to be revived, refreshed, transformed. If you are tired, you have been doing a lot of mental work, you may be tired, and not thinking correctly. You need your mind renewed.

Sleep and rest are needed. That is when your mind gets a chance to rest. Many people try to burn the candle at both ends. That expression means that they stay up late and get up early. They do not get enough sleep. Actually, your whole body suffers when you do that. God has designed your body to renew itself. Literally, cells are replaced as you sleep. However, it always starts at point A and works toward Z. So if you never get enough sleep, parts of your body never get refreshed.

A scripture for meditation for the health of your mind and soul is:

Ephesians 4:23 - and be renewed in the spirit of your mind,

October 7

You are the healed. Scripture tells you to let the redeemed say so. You are redeemed, all sickness, disease, illness, any of these are from the enemy. God has redeemed you. Galatians 3:13 tells you that you are redeemed from the curse of the law.

This means that whenever symptoms are attacking you, refuse them. You are the healed. You have the victory. You have already won.

Do I understand how bad you feel, how much you have tried, what the doctors say? Maybe not. I do know what the Bible says, and that is my final authority.

If you have been dwelling on how you feel, just realizing the truth of what the Bible says can be a powerful influence on your feelings.

Don't let your feelings dictate to you. You dictate to your feelings. You tell them to get in line with the Word of God. Speak to your body, your leg, your head, tell it to line up with the Word of God.

You may be surprised at how feelings will change when you do this.

> Psalm 107:2 - Let the redeemed of the LORD say so, whom He has redeemed from the hand of the enemy,

By Patricia L. Whipp

## October 8

When you are praying, for healing or anything else, you want your prayers to be heard. God answers all prayers that He hears. Scripture tells us that. (1 John 5:14) He doesn't hear any wicked, bad, wrong, evil thoughts. God has also told you not to grieve, some translations include that in the word iniquity.

Get yourself right with God, then pray for healing. If you are in grief, worry, sorrow, first seek God about that. Scripture tells you to cast your care on Jesus. (1Peter 5:7) Learn to do that. Trust that God will handle the problem. It may not be easy, but it is feasible to do these things. It is also very rewarding.

Casting your care on Jesus may be one of the hardest things some people will do. Learning to control thoughts has been a fight for me. Am I perfect in that area? No, but I'm much better.

These things will take you time to do. The day will probably come, you think you have learned. Then, a new season of learning more starts. After you learned to add, then you had to learn to multiply. The same thing is true with principles in the Bible.

Don't give up, don't quit. Be the victor God has designed you to be.

Psalm 66:18 - If I regard iniquity in my heart, the Lord will not hear.

## October 9

God wants long life for you. That is His plan for your life on this earth. He said that man's life was to be 120 years. (Genesis 6:3) Wouldn't you consider that to be a long life?

If God expects you to live 120 years, He certainly wants you healthy. Learning to walk in divine health is wisdom. When you are sick, you may not be as useful as when you are well.

Some illnesses are not serious. Someone who needs to wear glasses can be strong, wise, healthy in every way. God has given man the wisdom to design glasses.

Hearing aids are very developed today. Don't put someone down because they use hearing aids. I have heard ministers criticized for using doctors, glasses, or hearing aids.

Learn to not judge others. You are only to judge yourself. What others do, or need, is between them and God. Not you.

Man has developed many devices to aid people. This wisdom came from God. The earth suits that we wear have limitations. But learn to exercise your faith, to keep it in good working order, and be thankful for the wisdom that God has given people to aid problems.

> Psalm 91:16 - With long life I will satisfy him, and show him My salvation."

By Patricia L. Whipp

## October 10

God wants you healed. He asks that you serve Him. This was true in the Old Testament. As a child of God, He still wants you doing the thing He has asked of you.

Spend time praising God, thanking Him for His love, and for the things He does for you. The scripture below is good as a healing scripture, it is also a good scripture for when you pray over your food.

God will bless your bread and water. You want your food sanctified, you want it pure so that you don't get sick from the food you eat. You want your water pure.

If you pray this over your food, you not only are getting the food purified, you are getting your body cleansed. Sounds like an excellent scripture to keep in your frequently used file.

> Exodus 23:25 - "So you shall serve the LORD your God, and He will bless your bread and your water. And I will take sickness away from the midst of you.

## October 11

Do you know anyone who has a balance problem, someone who falls at times? This can be true of someone of any age, but the elderly are often susceptible to falling.

This does not have to be. If the cause of the problem is known, there may be scriptures dealing directly with the problem. But there are times when the true cause is not known. Doctors may have a theory, but they can't prove what they think is the problem.

Did you know that the angels will bear the person up so that they don't fall? There are also scriptures where God says He will hold you up.

Learn to draw from God, both directly and through the use of His angels. God has provided help for us, let's learn to take advantage of this help.

> Psalm 91:12 - In their hands they shall bear you up, lest you dash your foot against a stone.

## October 12

God wants you healed. He paid a terrible price for your healing. His first born son was beaten and died on a cross, that included your healing.

God has always wanted His people healed. When the Israelites were brought out of Egypt, God promised them that none of the diseases put on the Egyptians would be put on them. In fact, they were told that all sickness would be taken away.

Sickness is not of God, and never has He wanted His people to suffer. Sickness is from the enemy. There is nothing natural about sickness.

This includes old age, aging should not include sickness. You should have your strength and all movement. Learn to see yourself as God wants you, and as He sees you.

> Deuteronomy 7:15 - And the LORD will take away from you all sickness, and will afflict you with none of the terrible diseases of Egypt which you have known, but will lay them on all those who hate you.

October 13

Are you feeling weak? Are you stressed? The first thing to do is get rid of all cares, any unforgiveness. Give your cares to Jesus. He can handle them. You cannot.

If you are offended by anyone, not forgiving them only hurts you. It doesn't bother them at all. Check that out. How about the government? Are you offended at the government? You don't have to think something is right, just don't walk in offense. Try it. You will discover there is a difference. Forgive, let God lead you.

Spend time with God. Praise Him. Listen to praise music. Talk to God. Let God lead you in the steps you are to take. God will strengthen you. He will guide you. As your strength returns, you will feel much better. As you praise Him, your joy will build up and your strength will increase.

> Isaiah 40:31 - But those who wait on the LORD shall renew their strength; they shall mount up with wings like eagles, they shall run and not be weary, they shall walk and not faint.

By Patricia L. Whipp

## October 14

Jesus told us that we have authority over serpents, scorpions, and all power of the enemy. That means that is all under our feet.

The Amplified Bible includes physical and mental strength and ability over all the power of the enemy. When our minds grasp what Jesus has given us, we will shout for joy. We have the victory, we win. Nothing can defeat us.

Grasping these facts takes meditation, study, and faith in the Word of God. We have so much. Yesterday, the wind was taken out of my sails for a little while. It caused me to realize how much our emotions rule us. Once again the statement, "I am not moved by how I feel, I am only moved by what the Word of God tells me," came to mind.

It is so important to hold onto that decision. I sat and realized that my feelings can sure change quickly, and be so meaningless.

I suggest you state, out loud, "I am the healed and I am saying so."

> Luke 10:19 - Behold, I give you the authority to trample on serpents and scorpions, and over all the power of the enemy, and nothing shall by any means hurt you.

288

## October 15

God tells you that His Word is healing to you. The Hebrew word used actually means medicine. He tells you to listen to His sayings. He also says to keep them in front of your eyes. Many people just listen to teachings and the Bible, but they don't read it. You must do both.

Meditate includes in it's definition "to mutter." So, if you are meditating on a scripture, and you quote it out loud, you are listening to His scriptures.

But the scripture says, "Do not let them depart from your eyes." That is equally important as hearing the scriptures. It is very important to hear and to see the scriptures.

The scriptures are life, that means healing and health. It is as important to take scriptures as it is to take medicine. I would be inclined to say it may be more important to take scriptures, than it is medicine.

Proverbs 4:21 - Do not let them depart from your eyes; keep them in the midst of your heart;

## October 16

Have you heard people say things like, "The men in my family have always died young with heart attacks."? Or another one is, "The men in my family all go bald." These are sometimes called generational curses.

The word 'curse' fits well. They are all listed under the curses of the law. A good place to find most of the curses of the law is in the Book of Deuteronomy, chapter 28, verses 15-68.

Many things are included in there. But the good news is that Galatians 3:13 tells us that we are free from the curse of the law.

You don't have to be a victim of these problems. Even in the Old Testament, there are several places where God told the Jews that these curses did not apply to them. No one had to die for the sins of their parents.

Today, these are often called generational diseases. Once again, you have the right to be free from these. You have to claim your freedom. Let the enemy know you don't accept these problems. Take authority and claim your rights.

> Ezekiel 18:20 - The soul who sins shall die. The son shall not bear the guilt of the father, nor the father bear the guilt of the son. The righteousness of the righteous shall be upon himself, and the wickedness of the wicked shall be upon himself.

## October 17

God wants you healed. He sent Jesus for you, that you might have everlasting life. What did Jesus preach? Jesus preached that He had come to heal the brokenhearted. He also preached that He came to heal the sick.

God is not only interested in healing people who have a disease, or other sickness, He is interested in healing the brokenhearted. Your hurts are meaningful to God. He wants your soul healed as well as your body.

You will have different steps in healing the soul, but it can be healed quickly just like the body can.

God wants you healed, spirit, soul and body. He wants every part of you healed.

Learn to trust God. A major part of that trust is simply a decision. Just as salvation was a decision, agreeing to trust God is a decision. Make the choice today.

Be healed. Be whole. Be free from all sickness and disease.

Psalm 147:3 - He heals the broken-hearted and binds up their wounds.

By Patricia L. Whipp

## October 18

You must listen for the voice of God. You don't hear God with your physical ears, you hear Him with your spiritual ears. That is inside of you. That voice can be as loud to you as your physical voice is, or there may be no sound. You sense it.

Some people take years to start hearing that voice, others learn right away. Don't have thoughts about what you have to do, or how to hear. Relax, spend time worshiping God, seek Him with your heart, not your mind. He wants to talk to you. He wants you to talk to Him.

God wants you fellowshipping with Him. He also wants you healed. If you are seeking a healing, spend time worshiping God. Spend time talking to Him.

Sometimes your thoughts, your mind, can get in the way of your healing. Quiet those down, and let God spend time with you. You just might find you are healed when you are through!

> Exodus 15:26 - and said, "If you diligently heed the voice of the LORD your God and do what is right in His sight, give ear to His commandments and keep all His statutes, I will put none of the diseases on you which I have brought on the Egyptians. For I am the LORD who heals you.

## October 19

Do you say, "I get the flu every year."? Or do you say, "By His stripes I am healed."? Your head can cause you to get sick if you believe and speak the wrong report!

If the news is talking about the Whatsit Flu coming this winter, and the doctor says you had better get the flu shot, it is going to be an epidemic, do you agree?

What did God say? What does the Bible tell you? You have decisions to make. You have to decide what you believe, and what you need to do. If you don't believe the Bible, maybe you had better get that Whatsit Flu shot.

If you believe that the Bible is true, then you need to pray and ask God what you should do. God may tell you to go to the doctor. There is not enough time for your faith to work.

Do you see what an influence your mind is, and how much trouble you can get yourself into? Your tongue speaks what you are thinking. The enemy seeks to hurt you, he uses many ways.

This is why you must spend time in the Bible, meditating the Word, and in prayer. You do that so you can hear God's guidance.

> Psalm 71:24 - My tongue also shall talk of Your righteousness all the day long; for they are confounded, for they are brought to shame who seek my hurt.

By Patricia L. Whipp

## October 20

Do you feel run down, weak, you seem to have no energy? Then you need healing! It is very possible that it is not a physical healing that is needed. It could be in the soul. If you are depressed, stressed, or other mental problems, that could cause a lack of energy. God wants you healed. It doesn't matter if the problem is physical, or some other problem, God wants you well.

You need to seek God. If the problem is stress, your solution could be as simple as giving Him your cares. It could be that your Word level is low. Are you reading your Bible every day? Are you meditating on scriptures every day? What is your prayer level? You need to spend time in prayer, every day. Are you spending time praising God? He wants to fellowship with you.

None of these need to be lengthy times. They can be spread out during the day. Do a little of one or more of these before you go to work. Do some of this during lunch. Then finish your time with God at night.

If a doctor gives you medicine, you might have to take a pill 3 to 5 times a day. Take a scripture 3 to 5 times a day. Seek God and let Him strengthen you.

> 1 Chronicles 16:11 - Seek the LORD and His strength; seek His face evermore!

## October 21

God wants you well. That has been established. I had a nice, Christian lady ask me once how I expected to die if I didn't get sick and die.

It is sad that many Christians believe that. Yet, there are examples in the Bible of people dying without being sick.

This is why we want to learn to walk in divine health; to live a full life, be strong, and fulfill the call on our lives.

This concept is foreign to some, but it should not be. Paul said that he had a choice, and at one point he decided he needed to stay here to continue teaching people. This is what we need to get solid in our minds. We need to learn to change our thinking, to realize that we have choices, to live our lives to the best of our ability as God would have us live.

> Genesis 49:33 KJV - And when Jacob had made an end of commanding his sons, he gathered up his feet into the bed, and yielded up the ghost, and was gathered unto his people.

By Patricia L. Whipp

## October 22

Peter and John were going into the temple. There was a man at the gate called Beautiful who was lame. He was laid there daily to beg. As Peter saw him, he stopped and spoke to the man. Then Peter lifted him up, and as he lifted him, he was healed.

What did the man do? He started leaping, jumping, walking, and praising God. When we receive a healing, what should we do? We should jump for joy, we should shout, and we should praise God.

Don't ever forget healings that God has done for you. Praise God for the healing. That is a part of your testimony. Tell others what God has done for you. As you witness of these healings, it builds the faith of others to know that God will do the same thing for them.

God is not a respecter of people. He wants people healed, and He will heal all who will receive. Help others to believe, to build faith in God, to know and believe the goodness of God.

> Acts 3:8 - So he, leaping up, stood and walked and entered the temple with them—walking, leaping, and praising God.

October 23

Learning to walk in divine health is a good thing to do. Most people do not realize that, after the flood, God set the life span of man at 120 years. That is how long you can expect to live.

During the Exodus, as they left Egypt and before they reached the promised land, God became upset with man. He said that the older generation, those who were adults when they left, could not enter the promised land. So, during that time, their life span was limited to seventy, possibly eighty years.

However, after they entered the promised land, that was no longer in effect. This means that the life of man was once again raised to 120 years.

Few people reach that age today. The reason is they don't seek to walk in divine health. Many people would rather just enjoy life. More people are living longer today, but so many have mental problems. That is not God's best. Neither is it divine health.

Learn how to live a productive life, a life devoted to fulfilling your call, and enjoy your life.

> Genesis 6:3 - And the LORD said, "My Spirit shall not strive with man forever, for he is indeed flesh; yet his days shall be one hundred and twenty years."

By Patricia L. Whipp

## October 24

Do you pray over your food? I don't mean do you pray before you eat, pray that Aunt Nettie gets better, that Uncle Bill gets a job, and whatever else you can think of.

Do you pray about the food and over the food? First, you are told to thank God for every good thing, but, there is a much more important reason for praying over your food. It is made pure, sanctified by prayer. What does that mean?

If the food is getting rancid, and you pray scriptures over it, the food is made pure. You will not get food poisoning. You should always use scriptures when you pray over food. There are many scriptures where God tells you He will bless your food; He will sanctify your food. He also tells you that you can drink any deadly thing and it will not hurt you. You do not do this on purpose, you are not protected if you do this on purpose. If you are served something that you know nothing about, you are protected.

Always, at home, at a restaurant, at a friend's home, pray over the food. If the host does not pray scriptures over the food, then quietly do so. This is a way to stay well, a part of walking in divine health.

> 1 Timothy 4:4–5 - For every creature of God is good, and nothing is to be refused if it is received with thanksgiving; for it is sanctified by the word of God and prayer.

## October 25

Do you, or someone you are praying for, need a real miracle? Is something wrong that seems impossible to cure or fix? Are there deformities in the body that need to be corrected?

First, settle in your mind, there is nothing God cannot cure, heal, or correct. God formed man in the beginning. He knew you from before the foundations of time. He knows what the original design for you was, and it wasn't deformed or sick. If there was an accident which has caused the problems, God knows how to correct that.

The next thing to settle in your mind is that God wants you healed. God wants the best for you. A part of what Jesus did for us happened on the way to the cross. He was beaten. Every stripe He received was to pay for your healing, for your life here on earth.

What can you believe for? What can you set your faith for? God is a God of miracles. There are times when we limit God. We listen to others—doctors, friends, we hear their reports, and believe their reports.

Decide what you can believe for, and go for it. Pray. Get agreement. If you are in a place where you can do so, draw from the anointing, then stand firm. Believe.

> Jeremiah 32:27 - "Behold, I am the LORD, the God of all flesh. Is there anything too hard for Me?

By Patricia L. Whipp

## October 26

God wants you well. This is something that I have stated over and over. It is a matter of brain-washing, getting this information totally established in your mind.

It is so easy to question this fact. It is so easy to think, this time that is not true.

The other thought is, what is God trying to teach me? Is that why this is taking so long? Let's turn this around, "What can I learn at this time?" The problem is with you, not with God. So, take time to study, pray, and find out what is causing the delay.

God loves you. We don't always hear what He is trying to express to us. But if you will do the things suggested, study, pray, fast, you will receive the answer.

More than once I have turned on the TV and the minister teaching answers a question I have been trying to find. I don't mean I listened for an hour, I mean within five minutes of my turning the TV on, I have something I have been looking for. Relax, and trust God to get the answer to you.

> 3 John 2 - Beloved, I pray that you may prosper in all things and be in health, just as your soul prospers.

October 27

Do you pray for other people to receive healing? Do you lay hands on the sick? Jesus said that all believers should lay hands on the sick. Do you have a co-worker at the office with a headache? Offer to pray for that person.

Does the thought come to you, "What if they don't get well?" First of all, that is not your problem. You are not the healer. Second, healings don't always manifest immediately.

What if they do get healed immediately? Are you prepared to witness to them? Sometimes, you can witness immediately, normally you will sow a seed, or water a seed that someone else has sown.

I had one coworker come to a Bible study in my home, and he was born again as a result of something this simple.

Mark 16:18 - they will take up serpents; and if they drink anything deadly, it will by no means hurt them; they will lay hands on the sick, and they will recover."

## October 28

There were two blind men who followed Jesus, they were crying out, "Have mercy on us." They followed Jesus into the house.

Jesus asked them a question. He asked if they believed that He could do this. When they responded, "Yes," He then said, "According to your faith let it be to you."

Do not be timid. Seek Jesus. Seek healing. God wants you healed. If you apply your faith, God is pleased.

Stretch your faith. Start with small things and build your faith up. When I first started learning this, I read in a book that God heals headaches. At that time, I was on a prescription for headaches. I have not had a headache since then. I have had opportunities, but I take authority over it.

Be prepared to apply your faith for healing, trust God, and watch God heal you.

> Matthew 9:28–29
> 28 And when He had come into the house, the blind men came to Him. And Jesus said to them, "Do you believe that I am able to do this?" They said to Him, "Yes, Lord."
> 29 Then He touched their eyes, saying, "According to your faith let it be to you."

## October 29

Jesus sent his twelve disciples out to minister to other people. He gave them power and authority over all demons and to cure diseases. As a born-again Christian, you have the same authority. You have the right to pray for people. You have the ability to pray for the sick and watch them recover.

Pray for people. Pray for strangers. Pray for family. Pray for friends. If you are standing in a check out line and the person in front of you is coughing, or shows some other sign of being sick, offer to pray for them.

Usually that is easy. To me it is amazing how often people appreciate being prayed for, even when they tell you that they don't believe in God.

You don't have to do any more than that. You don't need permission to take authority over demons. You don't need to put up with bad behaviors in your presence.

Also, pray for Christians everywhere to start using their authority. Pray for people everywhere to be born again, healed and set free.

> Luke 9:1 - Then He called His twelve disciples together and gave them power and authority over all demons, and to cure diseases.

By Patricia L. Whipp

## October 30

Jesus went in to all the cities and villages. He taught them. He healed every sickness and every disease among the people.

You can't have any sickness or any disease that God won't heal. It may be a new sickness, it may be something totally new, but God will heal it. God wants us well more than we do. We will have, but learn to ignore even, a minor ache or pain. One that just pops up once in awhile, we tend to ignore. Even those minor seeming problems, God wants us totally well.

It is important that people learn that God wants them well. It is important that people learn what the Bible says. That is why the Bible tells us to renew our minds. That is why meditation is both in the Old and the New Testaments. We need to learn what is promised to us, both for our use, and so that we can tell others.

God loves you, so much that He sent His only begotten Son to earth for you.

> Matthew 9:35 - Then Jesus went about all the cities and villages, teaching in their synagogues, preaching the gospel of the kingdom, and healing every sickness and every disease among the people.

## October 31

How you talk can affect your health! The words you hear, the words others around you speak, can affect your health.

If you constantly hear negative words, it can cause stress, hurts, and that will definitely affect your health. If you are around negative people, forgive them, and learn to not accept the bad influence they could have on your health.

If you constantly talk about how bad things are, or how bad the people around you are, right now, determine to stop. Habits are not usually broken easily, or quickly, but with God's help and your determined efforts, you can change.

You need to renew your mind to think on the good, to learn to talk the good, to know the effects of the ways you have been thinking and talking.

You do this by finding scriptures about how you should think, and meditating on these scriptures. As you change your thinking, your talking will change.

> Proverbs 16:24 - Pleasant words are
> like a honeycomb, sweetness to the
> soul and health to the bones.

By Patricia L. Whipp

## November 1

There is nothing about you that is too small for God to help you with. This includes your health. If something draws your attention, irritates you, or causes you problems, God is capable and desires to help you.

All you have to do is believe that He is interested in the small details. If it is something like the fact that you are left handed, or one ear looks higher to you than the other, these may have caused emotional problems. An emotional problem can be as serious as a physical problem. Find scriptures about how much God loves you. Let the love of God heal these problems.

If you have a physical problem which is also a health issue, then you have scripture to base your prayer on. With scripture, you've got God's attention and His Word to command the needed healing.

God loves you with an everlasting love. He is available all the time. He will talk to you. The answer may not come instantly, but it will come.

> Psalm 138:8 - The LORD will perfect that which concerns me; Your mercy, O LORD, endures forever; do not forsake the works of Your hands.

## November 2

God so loved the world that He gave His Son that all might live. (John 3:16) God loves every person born in this world. He wants the best for everyone. If you have a child who has difficulty learning, start praying the scripture below over your child.

Actually, this scripture can be used by anyone. God will help people, He will give them knowledge and skill. If you are a student, you can use this scripture for yourself in your studying.

In teaching, I had two students who were considered to have mental problems. Both had their oxygen stopped as an infant long enough to affect the brain. Yet, both of these students could figure out problems in math better than many "normal" children.

I also worked with a similar man at a church. Once again, he could reason how to set things up better than many people. Don't overlook what a child can do. Encourage them and help them. Watch them improve with this encouragement.

> Daniel 1:17 - As for these four young men, God gave them knowledge and skill in all literature and wisdom; and Daniel had understanding in all visions and dreams.

## November 3

God has provided healing for you. He wants you healed. Has that been said before? Your mind needs to be brain washed with the Word of God until you will not think any other way. That needs to become your only thought concerning your health.

God knows the evils that are on earth, He knows the sicknesses that have prevailed here. He knows the pain, discomfort, and other problems involved with sickness. This is why He has provided healing for not only His people, but everyone who will receive.

Healing is a witnessing tool available for you to use. When people see that God does heal, that is often all they need to know—they then want to receive God as their Lord and Savior.

For the Christian, this is why meditating on one or more healing scriptures a day is an excellent preventative medication for you to take. It is much healthier than a flu shot, much better for you, and scriptures have no bad side effects.

> Psalm 30:2 - O LORD my God, I cried out to You, and You healed me.

## November 4

Do you find that there are some people that you pray for and they do not recover? Sometimes, people who know you well, possibly before you started studying the Bible and you learned that healing is available, may doubt that you are capable of praying for them.

Sometimes, the best you can do is try to show them the Word. I have been told that I talk about the Bible too much.

Don't let that stop you. Keep on. You may need to put your efforts in praying for them, not talking to them.

Don't feel that you are alone. The same thing happened to Jesus.

> Mark 6:5–6
> 5 Now He could do no mighty work there, except that He laid His hands on a few sick people and healed them.
> 6 And He marveled because of their unbelief. Then He went about the villages in a circuit, teaching.

## November 5

A woman who was not a Jew came to Jesus and asked Him to heal her daughter. He spoke in a way that to us today would sound very rude. It was more common to the region and the people of that day.

The woman responded very strongly. She said, "Even the dogs under the table eat the children's crumbs." She showed that she knew that healing was available for all. Even dogs could be healed, meaning non-Jews.

Jesus said that because she showed so much knowledge, in other words, because of the faith she showed, her daughter was healed.

God wants every one healed. He has made healing available for all people.

> Mark 7:28–30
> 28 And she answered and said to Him, "Yes, Lord, yet even the little dogs under the table eat from the children's crumbs."
> 29 Then He said to her, "For this saying go your way; the demon has gone out of your daughter."
> 30 And when she had come to her house, she found the demon gone out, and her daughter lying on the bed.

## November 6

The holidays are approaching. Not only do we have holidays approaching, but there are school breaks coming. People are shopping, decorating their homes, preparing for feasts and other activities.

This is the time of the year when families get together. For some people, this is not considered a good time, it is more like a duty than fun.

It is very important to protect your peace at this time of the year. Jesus gave you your peace. But even before that, God promised peace to the people when the commandments were given. If you will obey your God, you will walk in peace.

God has always made peace available. This says the sword will not go through your land. Not only are the holidays coming, but threats are coming.

Claim your freedom, do not give into anxiety and stress over any of this. Walk in peace. Do not fear during the day, nor at night. God will protect you.

> Leviticus 26:6 - I will give peace in the land, and you shall lie down, and none will make you afraid; I will rid the land of evil beasts, and the sword will not go through your land.

By Patricia L. Whipp

## November 7

When you are sick, often you don't feel strong, you are weak. You may feel faint and you may be weary. These are not good feelings. You can't get things done. You don't get work done.

There are times when your body has been pushed to the point of exhaustion. You do need to take care of your body, you do need to give it proper rest. You may not have a disease, but you are at a point that you can't do your work.

Where can you find strength? Wait upon the Lord. Spend some time resting, if needed spend some time sleeping. But then you definitely need to spend some time with God. Praise Him, worship Him. Thank Him for what He does for you.

As you wait on the Lord, your strength will be renewed. You will be able to go forward with strength. You will be physically rejuvenated, as well as mentally rejuvenated.

> Isaiah 40:28–29
> 28 Have you not known? Have you not heard? The everlasting God, the LORD, the Creator of the ends of the earth, neither faints nor is weary. His understanding is unsearchable.
> 29 He gives power to the weak, and to those who have no might He increases strength.

## November 8

People who are not Christians are under the law of sin and death. They have no special promises to stand on. They really have nothing to look forward to. They seek fun, good things, and a rich life. They have nothing to look forward to after death.

For the Christian, they can live free from the law of sin and death. Jesus paid the price for a good life on this earth. They have health, prosperity, and happiness all available to them. Certainly bad things happen. But they deal with those and push forward to the good.

The Christian knows that when they die, they are instantly present with the Lord. They were with God before they were born on earth, and they return to the Lord in heaven. How sweet is the sound of that.

This scripture below becomes a boost to your immune system. You are to be free from sickness. You are to be free from a lingering death. Jesus has set you free.

> Romans 8:2 - For the law of the Spirit of life in Christ Jesus has made me free from the law of sin and death.

By Patricia L. Whipp

## November 9

Healing can come in many different ways. At times, Jesus asked people to do different things to receive their healing. In the Old Testament, there were times when people were asked to do different things to receive their healing.

Definitely, if you apply your faith and pray, or are prayed for, healing is available. We know that, if we pray for anything which is God's will, it comes.

It is not always necessary for the person being prayed for to use their faith. We know that the Spirit gives some people gifts of healings. Those people, often in meetings, have a special gift, and anyone including non-believers gets healed. This can be as a sign to others. Also, the workings of miracles is another manifestation.

For a believer, setting your faith, letting it be in action in services where there are manifestations of the Spirit in action, is a powerful weapon against all illness.

> 1 Corinthians 12:7 - But the manifestation of the Spirit is given to each one for the profit of all:

## November 10

There are things that you can do to speed up your healing. These do not convince God that you should be healed. They help you to be prepared to trust and believe God.

One is to fast. This does not have to be a long fast, but fasting can be used to draw your attention to God. It is often mentioned in the scriptures, both the Old and the New Testaments.

When you are eating, many people tend to be more focused on their own body than on God. Often, you may eat too much at times, and then feel uncomfortable, and simply be very body minded.

Fasting does not have to be food. One person who used to teach that fasting was only food had God tell him to fast something else for a few days. You could fast TV for several days.

Seek God and see what He would have you do. Isaiah says that if you fast, your healing shall spring forth speedily.

> Isaiah 58:8 - Then your light shall break forth like the morning, your healing shall spring forth speedily, and your righteousness shall go before you; the glory of the LORD shall be your rear guard.

## November 11

Be sure you are walking in forgiveness. If you have someone, or something, you have not forgiven, you hinder your prayers. Your healing normally comes through prayers, so you also hinder your healing.

Something I just realized this year, are you angry with what a public figure has done? It could be a well known sports figure, a politician. Do you get upset every time you hear their name, or their latest story? Forgive!

This does not mean you have to like what they have done, but if you are getting upset, then you are not in forgiveness. No, you don't go to them and tell them, unless you know them. But you must forgive for your health's sake. Your blood pressure, stress, anxiety and much more are all at stake.

> Matthew 6:14–15
> 14 "For if you forgive men their trespasses, your heavenly Father will also forgive you.
> 15 But if you do not forgive men their trespasses, neither will your Father forgive your trespasses.

## November 12

Frequently, when I pray for someone, I have used two scriptures. One of those scriptures is Galatians 3:13 which says that you are redeemed from the curse of the law. The other one I use is Deuteronomy 28:61. That is a very generic scripture.

There are many diseases listed, not under today's names, but things like fever, plague, blindness, boils. Many things are listed under the curse of the law in Deuteronomy 28, but verse 61 covers everything. It says every sickness and every plague that isn't listed. This means that everything must be covered. It is either listed, or this verse covers it.

God is a good God. He didn't want people suffering sickness. That was never His intention, never His plan. That is why I like this combination of verses so much. It proves to us that God wants us well. Praise God for His goodness, and His mercy.

> Deuteronomy 28:61 - Also every sickness and every plague, which is not written in this Book of the Law, will the LORD bring upon you until you are destroyed.

> Galatians 3:13 - Christ has redeemed us from the curse of the law, having become a curse for us (for it is written, "Cursed is everyone who hangs on a tree"),

## November 13

God heals all of your diseases! Praise God for His goodness. Praise God for His healing. Don't ever think God has caused a disease you have. Don't ever think that He is delaying your healing.

God wants you healed. He wants every disease gone from your body. Sometimes, the healing of a disease is sped up. At other times, it takes its normal amount of time, but healing is promised.

The methods that are used will often vary. You can't expect the same results that Susie had, or that John had. Don't compare. You are a unique individual.

As you are believing for healing, keep your eyes on Jesus. Spend time in praise and worship. Know that healing is promised and don't be concerned about how.

Often, many people get caught up in logistics, wanting to know how, why, etc. The important thing is your healing, focus on Jesus and good health. Don't forget to say thank you for the healing.

> Psalm 103:3 - Who forgives all your iniquities, Who heals all your diseases,

# November 14

It is important to remain single minded. Once you pray for healing, your faith is set, don't look back, don't doubt, don't prepare for failure. God's Word promises victory. Keep your mind focused on your healing.

If you have an actual picture, for example, if you used to do gymnastics and your leg is broken, post a picture of yourself healed. Picture yourself doing the things you used to do again.

If you are believing for something where you don't have a picture of the healing in your mind, you need to develop that picture.

God gave you an imagination. That is built into you. You can picture in your mind the healing. As an example, if you are believing for healing for a child with crossed eyes, see that in your imagination. See that eye healed.

The Israelites constantly forgot the path. They were very double minded. Don't do as they did. Learn to be wise, learn to trust God, learn to follow His lead, to believe His Words.

> Psalm 107:43 - Whoever is wise will observe these things, and they will understand the lovingkindness of the LORD.

## November 15

When you have prayed for healing, it is good to find scriptures which give you a picture of yourself healed. You can use these to maintain your healing. If you do nothing, the enemy can bring your sickness right back on you.

Scriptures help you receive your healing. They help you maintain your healing, they help you to walk in divine health. Sounds to me like you always need scriptures. They are prevention, medicine, and maintenance.

You want to maintain your strength. The scripture below would also be useful for feet and legs. I am sure that you can find other uses for this scripture as well.

It is always good to have two to five scriptures that you are using. They can be different, but it is best if you know of other scriptures which show the same thing. There are places that say to have two or three witnesses. This can be two or three similar scriptures.

> Habakkuk 3:19 - The LORD God is my strength; He will make my feet like deer's feet, and He will make me walk on my high hills....

# November 16

You have seen people bent over. They can not straighten up. Their walking is awkward, some are bent clear over, some just a little bit. Then, usually their neck is bent because they hold their head up to see where they are going.

For someone with a hump on their back, that person also is often bent over because of the hump. Most often this occurs in women, but it can occur in a man as well.

God is as interested in that person's health as He is any other health problem. There was a description of this in Luke 13. What did Jesus do? He laid His hands on the woman and immediately she was made straight.

We have been given the same power today that Jesus had. God wants that person straightened up as much as He wants someone's fever gone. Don't be moved by a person's age or their appearance. If you are the person with a problem like that, pray. Believe God. There is a healing revival going on around the world, start being a part of it.

Get your healing, pray for others. If you have doubts, deal with those first. Get your mind renewed to know what is God's will. Believe, and be a part of the healing revival.

> Luke 13:13 - And He laid His hands on her, and immediately she was made straight, and glorified God.

## November 17

Job had learned that God was good. He taught others things God would do. His friends reminded Job of some of the things he had said. There is truth in these words, and this truth is supported elsewhere in the scriptures.

God will uphold you if you are stumbling. He will hold your hand, He will stop you from falling. If you will trust God, rely on Him, He will bear you up. God will strengthen the feeble knees. God wants you healed.

It has always been God's plan that you would be healthy and strong. Yes, there are things that you can do to take care of yourself. Wise eating and exercise are always advisable, but God does not expect you to spend hours a day on your body.

God wants you spending time with Him reading the Word, praising Him. He wants you doing basic maintenance on yourself. God will uphold you, He will strengthen your knees, if you will believe Him, trust Him, and allow Him to help you.

Many times people stop God with the words of their mouth. They speak the negative which gives place to the enemy. Speak the Word, live the Word, trust God, and receive your help.

Job 4:4 - Your words have upheld him who was stumbling, and you have strengthened the feeble knees;

# November 18

God wants you to have good sleep. Sleep is important to your health. Some people are working two and three jobs to make more money. They are staying up late to work, and getting up early to work.

Some people do this to play, if that is you, stop now.

For the person who is working extra to try and make more money for the family, you are risking your health to do this. What would happen if you get sick? Then, all your income will be gone.

Learn to trust God. He is interested in your health and your family. Learn what God says about your finances and follow God's plan. It may not be the way the world thinks, but it works.

Your health, your family, your life are worth learning what God says to do. When you put God in charge, you tell Him you will trust Him, and you let God take over. Your health will improve and your finances will improve.

How? I don't know how He does it, but I do know what the Word says, and I have watched it work many times.

> Psalm 127:2 - It is vain for you to rise up early, to sit up late, to eat the bread of sorrows; for so He gives His beloved sleep.

By Patricia L. Whipp

## November 19

Jesus is your shepherd. God has always looked out for His people. He wants them healed, well, and in the fold. Jesus is our example of this. He looks out for His people, He protects them.

As a shepherd, He not only oversees, but when a sheep is lost, He goes looking for it. He does His best to bring the sheep back to the fold, back to safety, back to the flock with the other sheep.

Jesus gave His life for your safety. He gave His body for your healing. As a shepherd would check a sheep for wounds and other health problems, so Jesus wants you healed. He wants your wounds cleaned and protected. He will clean your wounds and bind them up to protect them from getting worse.

Don't ever run from Jesus, turn to Jesus. Let Him be your shepherd. Let Him be your healer.

> Ezekiel 34:16 - "I will seek what was lost and bring back what was driven away, bind up the broken and strengthen what was sick; but I will destroy the fat and the strong, and feed them in judgment."

## November 20

If you are anxious, you are stressed and that affects your health. It is absolutely essential that you learn to cast your care onto Jesus. That is so easy to say. It is not easy to do.

For your health's sake, I would suggest meditating on scriptures about cares of this world, that Jesus will handle your cares. That needs to become so strong in your mind and spirit that when something happens, it is one of your first thoughts.

God's peace is yours. Jesus gave you His peace. It resides within you, but you have to let it have first place in you. You have to let it rise up. You have to learn to walk in His peace.

Once you start walking in His peace, then you have a guide available for you. Anytime that peace starts to lift, you know to check, find out what is wrong. When bad news comes, don't let it dominate you. Learn to walk in the peace of God, follow the peace.

> Philippians 4:6–7
> 6 Be anxious for nothing, but in everything by prayer and supplication, with thanksgiving, let your requests be made known to God;
> 7 and the peace of God, which surpasses all understanding, will guard your hearts and minds through Christ Jesus.

By Patricia L. Whipp

## November 21

Do you fear the name of God? That word fear does not mean a terror type of feeling. It means a reverence, a worshipful awe of God. Do you honor His name above all names in the world?

God expects reverence. He is love, He will do anything for you, but for His love, He reserves the right to be worshiped. He is your creator, He is your all in all, so for you to praise Him, and worship Him, is very little to give in return for what He does for you.

For those who do fear His name, healing arises, the Sun of Righteousness with healing in His wings. That healing is for you. That is one of God's many ways of giving to you.

Learn to spend time in praise and worship. Put on a CD and listen or sing with a praise and worship session. Tell God how much you love Him. Do this, and receive your healing.

If you prefer, sing to Him. Sing songs with the understanding, sing songs in the spirit. Worship God, tell Him of your love for Him. Worship the creator.

> Malachi 4:2 - But to you who fear My name the Sun of Righteousness shall arise with healing in His wings; and you shall go out and grow fat like stall-fed calves.

## November 22

The scripture below appears several times in the Bible. This can apply to different areas of your life. This says that Jesus will heal the brokenhearted. Forgiving someone will definitely speed up healing a broken heart.

The broken heart does need healing. A broken heart is often something that was done to you, forgiveness is needed and healing is needed. It could be a person—-friend, child, or spouse killed in an accident. There may be forgiveness needed, but healing is definitely needed.

A captive can be physically captive, or a kidnapped child. It can also be someone who is addicted to drugs. All are captives. God is interested in any area of captivity. He wants to see the captive set free, whether it is your own doing or a victim situation.

In every area, God is available to heal and to help with all solutions. Put God first, in prayer, in thought, and in any action you choose to do toward the solution.

> Isaiah 61:1 - "The Spirit of the Lord GOD is upon Me, because the LORD has anointed Me to preach good tidings to the poor; He has sent Me to heal the brokenhearted, to proclaim liberty to the captives, and the opening of the prison to those who are bound;

## November 23

Your soul encompasses your mind, your will and your emotions. Learning to renew your mind, to bring your will and emotions into subjection of the Bible, is a life long task. But the rewards of doing this are worth the efforts.

King David said that only because God was on their side did Israel escape being destroyed by the enemy. He says that their souls escaped as a bird from a snare. Many people would say the same thing today.

When you learn this, healing becomes more available. As you learn that God is on your side, that He wants you healed, then it becomes easier to believe God for that healing. This should help you to understand why I say to learn to walk in divine health. Meditating on scripture is the way you renew your mind. It is also a way to build a healed mentality into your mind.

This can be a part of walking in divine health. Just making a decision to put God first is a part of this as well. Make the choice to let God be first place in your life, and as you follow Him, you are on the road to divine health.

> Psalm 124:7 - Our soul has escaped as a bird from the snare of the fowlers; the snare is broken, and we have escaped.

# November 24

Maintain a healthy body. Learn to walk in peace, with no stress. Learn to be calm. You do not do any of this on your own. If you have bills due, you will be stressed. Even if someone is claiming you owe them money when you don't, you may be stressed.

The only way that you will learn to walk in peace, the only way you can avoid stress, is through God. Meditate God's Word, get it built into your mind and your spirit. You have to choose to trust God. You have to choose to believe Him.

When you do these things, the peace comes. Jesus gave you His peace, but you have to choose to walk in that peace. God promised to meet your needs, but you have to choose to walk in that lifestyle. You choose to trust God.

These things do not just fall on you. You work to bring them to you. How do you work? By being a doer of the Word, by meditating the Word, by keeping the Word before you night and day. The scripture below is good for this.

This is how you learn to walk in divine health, to walk in an abundant life. Jesus came that you might do these things.

> Psalm 85:8–9
> 8 I will hear what God the LORD will speak, for He will speak peace to His people and to His saints; but let them not turn back to folly.
> 9 Surely His salvation is near to those who fear Him, that glory may dwell in our land.

By Patricia L. Whipp

## November 25

Part of the lessons learned in healing are learning to live long, and to walk in divine health during your long life. Why should you want to live long, isn't it better to be in heaven?

Staying on earth is not a selfish act, it is to help others. To let others know about God, to witness to friends and strangers. You can witness in stores, on the sidewalk, at the bus stop.

When you let God be your source, then you can have more time to tell others about God. God is good. He does good things for His children. These good things can range from saving the best parking space for you, to supplying money to you. God is good.

God will lead you in the way you should go. He will direct you to find the things you need. He has provided peace for you, learn to walk the way God wants you to walk. Learn to do the things He wants you to do.

> Psalm 103:5 - Who satisfies your mouth with good things, so that your youth is renewed like the eagle's.

## November 26

Is there a sparkle in your eyes? If Jesus is your Lord and Savior, let the world know. Let the light shine out of your eyes. Let others see that something is different in you. Notice people's eyes. Watch for life. Your eye is the window through which they see what is in you.

Do you know that a good report, or good news, can make your bones healthy? Many translations use the word "fat" instead of healthy. You want your bones fat! You don't want them so thin that they become brittle. When they are brittle, you are not as healthy as when they are fat.

Brittle bones are apt to break. No more ice skating or roller skating when your bones are brittle. Falls are not good for brittle bones.

Learn to speak the good, to listen to the good. Do you have friends who always talk bad news? You might not want to be around them too much any more. You want to hear the good news.

> Proverbs 15:30 - The light of the eyes rejoices the heart, and a good report makes the bones healthy.

By Patricia L. Whipp

## November 27

Do you have a problem that causes you to stumble or fall? There are several scriptures where it says God will hold you up, He holds you with His hand. You should have prayed for your total healing, but as it comes, you don't want to fall. You could get hurt.

What is confidence? It is the full belief that the person, or thing, is fully capable of doing what it says. For example, if you are carrying a 100 pound box up a ladder, and the ladder says it will support up to 300 pounds, then are you fully confident that ladder will not fail? If God tells you He will do something, are you fully confident that He will do it?

The Bible says that the Lord is your confidence, that He will keep your foot from being caught! This is a scripture you can pray, and trust that God will protect you as you are walking.

What do you do with scriptures like these? Read them out loud to yourself. Faith comes by hearing. This is a form of meditation. Also, praise God for your complete recovery, so that the stumbling and falling is no longer a problem or concern.

> Proverbs 3:26 - For the LORD will be your confidence, and will keep your foot from being caught.

## November 28

Are you eating well? Do you have good choices available to you? Once again, your food is important to your health. Many people are growing their own food today. This gives you access to some ways to get better food.

The scripture below says if you are willing and obedient…. Doesn't this sound like you must make God first place in your life? This also lines up with, "Seek ye first…." (Matthew 6:33) Learn to make God your source, and put Him first in your life.

Being willing is listed first. This means that you must make the choice to put God first. It is a decision, then once you make the decision, you must be obedient. Be obedient to the will of God. Be obedient to the Word of God, and be a doer of the Word.

Make these choices, follow these actions, and you shall eat the good of the land. This will keep you healthier, happier, and more active.

> Isaiah 1:19 - If you are willing and obedient, you shall eat the good of the land;

## November 29

God loves you with an everlasting love. He wants you healthy, enjoying life, having fun, and doing work that He has for you. He has also designed you for the work He has for you.

Some people like to do repetitive things. Others get bored very quickly. If you are bored or unhappy, maybe you are doing it wrong, or maybe you are not in the right job. It can seem like an affliction to be in the wrong job!

Often, the word affliction is going to refer to pain, sickness, disease or other things related to your health. It can refer to your mental health as well as your physical health.

God wants you healed, both physically and mentally. This scripture tells you that God has delivered you out of your afflictions. Find several healing scriptures that speak to you, and meditate on those.

Why do I keep saying this? Because that is what the Bible tells us to do. This helps you to keep your mind focused on God, and to not be focusing on the world's way of doing things.

God's ways are healthy, fun, and a blessing for you.

> Psalm 34:19 - Many are the afflictions of the righteous, but the LORD delivers him out of them all.

## November 30

Do you feel healthy? Are you strong? God is the source for your health and your strength. God wants you healthy and He wants you strong. What is a good example to prove that to you?

When God took the Israelites out of Egypt, not one person was sick. These people had been slaves that were treated very poorly. They were not well fed.

Do you think that none were sick before the Passover? That seems impossible. They ate the Passover lamb. The Passover for the Israelites was the same as communion for the Christian. One of the benefits of communion is healing. Jesus was beaten for our healing.

It would seem that, with the first Passover lamb, all of the Israelites were healed. They were made ready for the forty year journey. The sicknesses that are recorded during the forty years all received healing.

God has never changed. He has provided healing for you, and wants you to partake of this healing. Look to Jesus and trust Him for your healing and divine health.

> Psalm 62:7 - In God is my salvation and my glory; the rock of my strength, and my refuge, is in God.

# December 1

There is no healing that is too hard for God. God will heal anyone and anything. When the crowds followed Jesus, the multitude brought the lame, blind, mute, maimed and others. None of these were too hard for Jesus.

Is deliverance needed? That never stopped Jesus. He wondered at the unbelief of His disciples that it defied them.

Jesus told His disciples that when He was gone, they would do greater works than what He had done. I've heard many explanations of what that meant. Some of them seemed to me to be pretty wild. Basically the person didn't believe that Jesus meant what He said.

We need to learn to believe the Bible. There is a healing revival going on around the world. Much of this revival is going on outside of America, but it is here, it is coming. Start believing, start praying, and watch this revival come to your city.

You do not usually see these things on the daily news, however, look on the internet.

Pray, believe God, and you will be an important part of this revival.

> Matthew 15:30 - Then great multitudes came to Him, having with them the lame, blind, mute, maimed, and many others; and they laid them down at Jesus' feet, and He healed them.

## December 2

God has given you armor for your life on this earth. This armor helps you in every area of your life. That includes your health. It gives you strength, ways to maintain your health, ways to receive healing.

The world has weird ideas of what is truth. Many people have been taught in school some very false ideas of the word truth. Jesus brought us truth. God's Word is truth. (John 17:17)

This is why it is so important to learn what the Bible teaches. It is so necessary to know what is right and what is wrong. The idea, "If it feels good, if it feels right, do it," is what has led to some very false beliefs. If you have no idea of what is good, you can end up with very wrong thinking using that philosophy.

Strengthen your loins. Strengthen your whole body. Learn to walk in truth, in knowledge of the Word of God. Be born again, then you will have the right to the breastplate of righteousness. Walk with your armor on.

> Ephesians 6:14 - Stand therefore, having girded your waist with truth, having put on the breastplate of righteousness,

By Patricia L. Whipp

## December 3

Panic attacks are not fun. When someone experiences one, they are often in so much fear that they cannot easily be calmed down. Or possibly the person is practically frozen with fear and does not move much.

People of God are told not to be afraid of sudden terror, nor of trouble from the wicked. For a Christian, this is even stronger than in the Old Testament. A Christian has authority over many things.

Have you noticed that, with the shootings of Christians in other countries, there are no reports of anyone denying Jesus? When I have been in danger, which has only happened on the freeway, God usually has me wrapped in a blanket of peace. I have no other way to describe it.

Because of my experiences, it seems to me that God holds those people very closely. He must give them so much peace that they focus on the peace, not the threats. Learn to walk closely with God, and let His peace reign in your life.

Meditating on scriptures like the one below, building these into your mind and your spirit, will help you if you are ever in a threatening situation.

> Proverbs 3:25 - Do not be afraid of sudden terror, nor of trouble from the wicked when it comes;

# December 4

Healing is available today for anyone. Some people say that when Jesus died, healing ceased to be available. I have also heard it said that, when the last apostle died, healing ceased.

There are still apostles today. There are people who are ordained as apostles, and there are people who function as an apostle without the title. An apostle is someone who starts churches.

We see in Acts that Paul laid hands on Publius who was sick with a fever and dysentery. That man was healed instantly. That same anointing is available today. There are other scriptures where Jesus told you anyone who is born again can lay hands on the sick, and Jesus said they shall recover.

In Jesus' last words before He rose to sit at the right hand of the Father, He said, "Go… lay hands on the sick, and they shall recover." (Mark 16:18) You are to function as Paul functioned in this area of Jesus' ministry. Lay hands on the sick, and they shall recover.

You are not the healer, Jesus is. You are the ambassador, follow the instructions of Jesus.

> Acts 28:8 - And it happened that the father of Publius lay sick of a fever and dysentery. Paul went in to him and prayed, and he laid his hands on him and healed him.

## December 5

There are times when people are actually driven by a demon. Some diseases cause a person to have seizures. At times, that is caused by a demonic spirit, but not always. This is where it becomes important to learn to hear God.

What you do one time does not determine what you will do the next time. You can lay hands on the sick, pray for them, and watch them get well. In the example below, that would not have worked.

Don't let this example stop you from laying hands on the sick. Let it cause you to learn more, to learn to listen to the spirit, and to follow the leadings of the spirit. Let it be an inspiration for you to learn and to grow in the things of God.

> Mark 9:25–27
> 25 When Jesus saw that the people came running together, He rebuked the unclean spirit, saying to it, "Deaf and dumb spirit, I command you, come out of him and enter him no more!"
> 26 Then the spirit cried out, convulsed him greatly, and came out of him. And he became as one dead, so that many said, "He is dead."
> 27 But Jesus took him by the hand and lifted him up, and he arose.

## December 6

Walking in stress, anxiety, or any kind of fear is not good for you. It can cause all kinds of sickness and disease in your body. It can damage your heart. It is not good for your health in any way.

The world teaches you to learn to handle stress. The world says stress is normal, you have to learn to control stress. That is not what the Bible teaches. The Bible teaches you to trust God. Let Jesus have your worries. Let Him handle your cares.

Who designed you? God did. Who knows the most about how your body should work? God does. So, should you believe what the world says? Or should you believe what the Bible tells you?

It may seem too hard to do at first, but the benefits of trusting God are peace, calm, joy, quiet. In fact, there are many more benefits. Start today! Seek God first, hand your cares to Him, and enjoy your life.

> John 16:33 - These things I have spoken to you, that in Me you may have peace. In the world you will have tribulation; but be of good cheer, I have overcome the world."

## December 7

Sleep, rest and peace are all important to good health. If you don't have enough sleep and rest you will wear out, literally! Your body functions best when you are well rested.

Without peace, you are looking at anxiety, stress, and other problems that will cause you trouble. Anxiety and stress can kill you if you give them enough time in your body. They wear your body out.

Spend time with God. Get to know Him. Spend time reading the Bible. Spend time in prayer. Spend time meditating the Word. These are all things that you are told to do, and they will help you to learn more about God, to learn more of the blessings He has for you. Peace and good sleep can be blessings.

God has given you peace. He will give you sleep. God will protect you and keep you in safety. Learn to trust God, spend time with Him so that you may be in peace and sleep well. If you let anxiety keep you awake, you are missing a blessing God has for you.

Psalm 4:8 - I will both lie down in peace, and sleep; for You alone, O LORD, make me dwell in safety.

## December 8

Getting healed and walking in divine health all include eating well. The word in this Bible that is translated "the poor," normally means just that, but anyone could be applied to this verse.

God says you will eat and be satisfied. That word "satisfied" has several meanings. Full is one of them. It can also mean enriched or safe. If you are eating things that will make you sick, or that will not satisfy your whole body, or does not have proper nourishment for your whole body, then your body is not satisfied.

For some people, this may be because of a lack of money. Some foods cost more than others, so if you are not buying enough of what your body needs due to a lack of money, God says good foods will be available for you.

If you are eating poorly because that is what you like best, you need to make some changes in your lifestyle.

It also says to seek the Lord and praise Him. You can find things on the internet to support many different food styles. Seek God. He will guide you to what you need. Praise God, seek Him for help.

> Psalm 22:26 - The poor shall eat and be satisfied; those who seek Him will praise the LORD. Let your heart live forever!

## December 9

Have you prayed for a healing, received it, and you are waiting? Keep your hope in place, keep your faith set. This means you also keep your confession in line with the Word. You are healed.

You are not lying, you are following the Word. Stand strong. God is there, as you stand He will strengthen your heart. Sometimes things do take time. When a broken bone is set, it takes around 5 or 6 weeks to heal. Sometimes God speeds it up so fast it seems to be immediately, sometimes it takes a week. Time is really not important. It just seems like it is.

For people who are believing for a problem with their heart, this scripture is a good one to confess. It's good for anything, but your ears hear that God strengthens your heart, your heart hears it and perks up.

I know somebody who had heart problems. She confessed, did all the right things, also continued with what the doctor said to do. Now she has a new heart! The doctor was amazed, he ran a normal test, and said no one with the condition she had could possibly come out that strong on the test he ran. Praise God for His healing.

> Psalm 27:14 - Wait on the LORD; be of good courage, and He shall strengthen your heart; wait, I say, on the LORD!

## December 10

Do you, or someone you know, have a mental disorder? Autism is something that is becoming more widespread. There are definitely levels of this disorder, ranging from mild to severe.

If you have an autistic child, there can be many causes. The cause does not matter, God can cure anything. Some people have successfully used diet to control this disease. Not all cases are the same.

What is the same is that they are all under the curse of the law. God wants all people with mental problems set free. Scripture and prayer has a healing effect on all of these. This is what is known.

The scripture below is one that I know some use for their autistic child, that the child's mind will become normal; that the child will function with others, and be able to praise and glorify God with others.

The victory is yours, God wants you free. Pray, believe, and watch the healing manifest.

> Romans 15:6 - that you may with one mind and one mouth glorify the God and Father of our Lord Jesus Christ.

By Patricia L. Whipp

# December 11

Do you, or does someone you know, want a child and they have had difficulty having a child? That is under the curse. God wants you to have children. He has promised children to you. Children are a blessing and are promised.

There are many areas that we are robbed. Childbirth is one where people have been robbed. Do not be discouraged. There is nothing wrong with adoption. There are children that need to be adopted.

But if you want a child of your own, know that God has promised it to you. Abraham is an example of God fulfilling a promise of a child. John the Baptist is another miracle baby. His mother, Elizabeth, was past the time of childbearing.

If you are in a position of wanting a child, seek God, pray, find scriptures that support your desire. There are many. Meditate on these scriptures.

God loves you and wants the best for you.

Exodus 23:26 - No one shall suffer miscarriage or be barren in your land; I will fulfill the number of your days.

# December 12

Do you feel weak? God will strengthen you. There are many scriptures that tell you God is your strength, He will give you strength. The one below is talking about times when you need to protect your land.

You may ask, "How can I say 'I am strong'?" You can say that because you know God is strengthening you. If you have set your faith, you may be calling those things which be not as if they are. You are talking the way God wants you to talk.

The world's way of doing things is to wait until they manifest to say something. God's way is to speak something and watch it come to pass. God spoke everything we know into existence.

We are His children. He wants us doing the same thing. Your best way to do this is to find scriptures which support what you are believing for. Meditate on those scriptures. Pray for what you are believing, then speak them into existence.

Haven't you noticed children copy their parents? They copy their bad habits as well as their good habits. You are a child of God. Learn to behave as your Father wants you to behave.

> Joel 3:10 - Beat your plowshares into swords and your pruning hooks into spears; let the weak say, 'I am strong.' "

## December 13

The real you is a spirit! You are a spirit, you have a soul (mind, will, and emotions), and you live in a body. Your body is really your earth suit. Just like astronauts need a space suit, you need an earth suit when you are on earth.

When the body dies, it stays on earth, and the spirit is instantly with God in heaven. Many times people have been revived, or brought back to life. Their spirit is called back from heaven. There are people alive who can tell you their experiences in heaven before they were brought back to life.

In the scripture below, the man fell three stories. That was enough for serious injuries to the body. But when Paul felt life in him, there is no mention of other problems. He was fine.

You have the right to call somebody back to life, or to let them enjoy their new life in heaven.

> Acts 20:9-10
> 9 And in a window sat a certain young man named Eutychus, who was sinking into a deep sleep. He was overcome by sleep; and as Paul continued speaking, he fell down from the third story and was taken up dead.
> 10 But Paul went down, fell on him, and embracing him said, "Do not trouble yourselves, for his life is in him."

## December 14

This is a season to be merry, to have fun, and be joyful. Not everyone joins in. Some don't join in because of their beliefs. Others don't join in because of illness. They are oppressed, maybe depressed.

God wants you free from the oppressor. That is a mental condition that is certainly under the curse. You have every right to be free from the mental disorders. He wants you free from depression.

Did you lose a spouse, a child, or a close friend? These are all things that can be very upsetting, but God can heal this. You will need to be willing to let go of this, but when you learn what God has for you, when you realize long term grief is not of God, but is of the enemy, you are a step closer to freedom.

God says He will break in pieces the oppressor. That means your enemy will be broken in pieces. Take joy in the fact that God will have the final say. Have faith in God.

Trust God, let Him help you, and learn to walk in the joy and peace that He has for you.

> Psalm 72:4 - He will bring justice to
> the poor of the people; He will save
> the children of the needy, and will
> break in pieces the oppressor.

## December 15

Often when you are sick you feel weak, and cannot do much. Having strength and power is very helpful. God has strength and power. He wants you well, He wants you strong. As you get well, you feel your strength return.

God loves you very much, Jesus gave His life for you, the desire is for your way to be perfect, not sickly. Hold onto those thoughts. This is a good scripture to use, to see in your mind.

Who wants you sick? The devil. Who wants you well? God. God is the healer. You live in a world that is being contaminated and actually being destroyed by an enemy. His time to be here is short, then there will be no sickness.

During your time on this earth, healing is provided. Don't forget that. Healing is available. It is for you, your family, and your friends. You are to live in health, and you are to pray for others, that they might live in health.

Go into all the world, that can be next door, tell them your story, how you came to know Jesus. Tell them of the goodness of God, and pray for the sick that they might recover.

> 2 Samuel 22:33 - God is my strength and power, and He makes my way perfect.

## December 16

Many scriptures throughout the Bible refer to both eyes and ears. God wants you to be able to see well, and to hear well. Does that hearing always refer to the physical ear? At times, it can refer to the spiritual ears.

You want to hear the Holy Spirit when He talks to you. He brings you messages from God. He lets you know what God wants you to know at that time. This verse can definitely be used for hearing the Holy Spirit.

The Hebrew word used which is translated dim can also mean not looking or closed. Are you looking away from what God wants you to see? Are you not looking in the direction He wants you to look? This scripture can be used for what the Spirit is showing you.

This scripture can also be used for your physical eyes and your physical ears. Are you not seeing as you should, not hearing as you should? God wants your physical eyes open, He has things to show you. He wants your physical ears hearing. He has things for you to hear. God will show you things for you to do, and He wants you hearing some things. Enjoy this verse, and meditate on it for many purposes.

Proverbs 20:12 - The hearing ear and the seeing eye, the LORD has made them both.

## December 17

Have you heard about the woman with the issue of blood in the Bible? Jesus healed that woman. Doctors could not do that. She had spent all of her money on doctors, but they could not heal her.

There were several blind men mentioned in the Bible. There was nothing that man could do to help them see. All that were mentioned during the life of Jesus were healed. Jesus was able to heal them.

There was a man who had a withered hand, Jesus healed him. Jesus made his withered hand straight like the good hand. Man cannot do that, but Jesus can and did.

There were several places when Jesus was working with the multitudes that the maimed, the blind, the deaf, all sick were healed. Many of these the medical profession cannot do anything about, but Jesus can.

What do you need healing from? There is nothing impossible for God. He still heals today. He heals through doctors, He heals through churches, He is available and will heal all that believe Him.

> Mark 9:23 - Jesus said to him, "If you can believe, all things are possible to him who believes."

# December 18

This is the season known for peace. God has given us year-round peace, but even non-Christians know this season as one of peace. This is a time you can talk about the peace of God to others easier than any other time in the year.

Do you know what peace means to your body? If anyone is sick, if they will stay in peace, their healing can come much faster. The peace helps the body to recover.

So often with a serious illness, such as cancer, many people become stressed and anxious. These factors alone can make you sick. They cause conditions and release hormones into the body that can cause illness.

Learn to trust God, to believe that He wants you well, to walk in peace.

If there is fear in you, that is not of God. Speak to the fear and tell it to leave. You have the authority to do this. When you do this in faith and trust, it must leave.

Let joy rise up in you. There is peace in you, Jesus gave it to you. Just as you can speak to fear and tell it to leave, you can speak to peace and tell it to rise up. Call forth the peace and enjoy.

> 2 Thessalonians 3:16 - Now may the Lord of peace Himself give you peace always in every way. The Lord be with you all.

# December 19

God has always wanted His people well. When the Israelites were restored, one of the things which God said about them is in the verse below; God will heal you and reveal abundance of peace and truth.

God wants this plus more for His church. You are children of God. He wants every person healed. He wants every person walking in peace. He wants every person walking in truth.

That is what God wants for you.

You have a role to play in these being accomplished. God will do things a few times for you, but you are expected to grow and to do things yourself. You are expected to apply your faith for your healing.

Jesus gave you His peace, but you need to take steps to walk in peace. You need to learn to walk in peace. You can block peace if you pick up cares, if you pick up worry and stress. You have a role to play in walking in peace.

God's Word is truth. You are expected to get into the Word, study, meditate, and learn what God has for you. God wants you to have these things, don't block them.

> Jeremiah 33:6 - Behold, I will bring it health and healing; I will heal them and reveal to them the abundance of peace and truth.

## December 20

The holidays are here. We have Thanksgiving, followed by Christmas, and then New Years. I would say that is a lot of feasting, food, drinking, and more food. There are very few people that do not party at least a few days throughout this season.

God established feasts. He designed feasts. He expects us to have fun and to enjoy ourselves. Even with this, He also expects us to use wisdom, restraint, and to be a witness to others.

You can have a good time. If you indulge moderately, if you are not vulgar with your talk, there is nothing to be concerned about. Both your health and your witness are things you need to be aware of, and to be wise.

Some people want to forget their health totally. That is not wisdom. Most people would say their witness to others is important, but they forget that and don't practice what they say.

Have fun at the parties, and at the family gatherings. Remember to walk in peace and joy. Don't forget that you are a child of God.

Romans 14:17 - for the kingdom of God is not eating and drinking, but righteousness and peace and joy in the Holy Spirit.

By Patricia L. Whipp

## December 21

Christmas time should be a time of peace. Many people send out Christmas cards which say "Peace" on them. Yet, are you walking in peace? Are you busy, stressed, trying to get things done? Do you know what that does to your health?

Stress, worry, cares, are all things which badly affect your health. Your heart does not handle stress well. Your body as a whole is tensed up. Your body does not handle stress well. Learn to walk in peace.

Do your body and yourself a favor. Find some scriptures on peace, and quote them out loud daily for awhile. By awhile, I mean a week, maybe a month. Practice settling down, putting aside stressful situations. Give the problems to Jesus. He said He would take them.

Then spend time in praise and worship, listening to music, talking to God, being restful. Don't have time? You have to put some things aside, don't do them, and put God first. Ask God what you can skip, or how you can do them. He will help you.

> Jeremiah 29:11 - For I know the thoughts that I think toward you, says the LORD, thoughts of peace and not of evil, to give you a future and a hope.

# December 22

The Greek word used for sanctify can mean to purify. It can refer to spirit, soul, or body. If your body is purified, all sickness and disease would have to leave! Having your mind or soul purified would be to get rid of bad thoughts.

That could be a Christmas present for yourself. It is something that you can pray for others, but you can't do it for them. You would need to spend time in prayer with God and in the Word!

This is one of the reasons it is so necessary to spend time reading the Bible. Everyday! It is also helpful to find some scriptures that say what you want to accomplish for yourself and spend time meditating on those.

The verse listed below says it all. It tells you that you are sanctified by the truth. Then it tells you that the Bible is truth. We have other scriptures that tell us that the Word is healing to our flesh.

Don't ever get so busy that you can't spend a few minutes in the Word. Look for ways to find more time every day in the Word. This can be a few minutes, several times a day.

Praise God, worship God, tell Him that you love Him. Read His Word, meditate on His Word.

John 17:17 - Sanctify them by Your truth. Your Word is truth.

## December 23

Do you, or someone you know, have problems with memory? This could be anyone, from a child trying to learn their multiplication tables to a senior who is forgetting things, and is frustrated over this.

This is a health issue, as much as any other sickness. Start with scriptures. You want a scripture which will cause your mind, your memory, to be renewed. You are also feeding your spirit with scripture.

The scripture below says, "I will not forget your Word." As you get that built into your memory, it helps your memory to remember. I will not forget.... From that you can transfer to multiplication tables, or anything else you need to memorize. Chemistry charts?

The Word is medicine to the body. Your mind is housed in your brain which is part of your body. So, this becomes healing to your memory.

Will this work with general forgetfulness? Certainly. God's Word is health, it is medicine, it strengthens, and it heals.

> Psalm 119:16 - I will delight myself in Your statutes; I will not forget Your Word.

## December 24

Good scriptures to meditate for healing include not only traditional healing scriptures, but scriptures that give you a visual of you being healed. When you meditate scriptures, you are feeding your mind, your spirit, and giving medicine to your body.

Do you, or someone you know, have problems with your neck? Maybe you can't turn your head easily, maybe your neck hurts. The scripture below refers to your head being lifted up. What lifts your head up? Your neck, this is a good visual for your neck.

God accepts sacrifices that are offered to bless Him. A sacrifice of joy is a good way to bless God. Jump, dance, sing for joy. This blesses God, and is strength to your body. Sing praises to God. He is blessed by praises.

Lift your head up, praise the Lord, and let God shower blessings down on you.

> Psalm 27:6 - And now my head shall be lifted up above my enemies all around me; therefore I will offer sacrifices of joy in His tabernacle; I will sing, yes, I will sing praises to the LORD.

By Patricia L. Whipp

## December 25

In the beginning the Word was with God. Revelations says His name is called "The Word of God." (Revelations 19:13)

Jesus was sent to the earth to redeem man. In the process of doing this, many provisions were made available for man here on earth. One of these is healing.

At His death, Jesus was beaten before He was hung on the cross. By the stripes on His back, your healing was paid for. It has been bought for you. There are several scriptures which tell you this.

Also, in Psalms it says, "He sent His Word, and healed them...." (Psalm 107:20) You are healed by the stripes of Jesus, and you are healed by the Word of God. (Proverbs 4:20-23)

At times, I ponder what the Jews felt these scriptures meant. They knew healing was available, but the fullness of these scriptures was not available and had not been revealed yet.

As revelation knowledge increases, we learn much more, and will see much more, about the healings that are available and will be accomplished in the days ahead.

> John 1:1 - In the beginning was the
> Word, and the Word was with God,
> and the Word was God.

## December 26

Nothing is impossible with God. He can heal anything. When the doctors tell you that they can do nothing, you know a God who can heal anything. When the doctors tell you something is impossible, you know a God who says, "With God all things are possible."

I am not saying don't go to a doctor. There are times when God wants to use the doctors. Don't stay away from doctors because you heard a minister that does not go to doctors. You hear God. When he says go, you go. Many times God wants to heal you. You will have a witness to not go to the doctor at that time.

However, when the doctor says that it is impossible, don't give up. God can step in and take over.

There are times, for example, if an appendix bursts, there may not be time to activate your faith. You could be dead very quickly if you don't use a doctor.

Don't go to a doctor without activating your faith. God can do miracles with a doctor.

Do not ever give up, and do not ever forget, with God all things are possible.

> Matthew 19:26 - But Jesus looked at them and said to them, "With men this is impossible, but with God all things are possible."

By Patricia L. Whipp

## December 27

God is no respecter of people. What He does for one person He will do for another. Not everyone is beautiful in the worldly sense. But everyone is beautiful to God. If you don't like your looks, seek God. He can help you.

Sometimes, there are accidents, and a scar appears. There are diseases that cause things not to look right. Any disease can be healed. The residue of the disease may leave a blemish. Seek God. Some things doctors can fix, most things God will fix.

My hands have blemishes. I have started praying and, in some areas, I have seen definite improvement. Learn to thank God for every improvement, and not be disappointed when some things take more time than others.

Learn to be moved only by the Word. Do not let negative comments from others disturb you. Easier said than done, but start putting God first, trust Him, and watch Him cause changes on you. Meditate the scripture below. Pull the parts of it you need into your self image.

> 2 Samuel 14:25 - Now in all Israel there was no one who was praised as much as Absalom for his good looks. From the sole of his foot to the crown of his head there was no blemish in him.

# December 28

You want to have a strong heart. You want to have good courage. No matter what is happening, God will protect you. If you have heart problems, God can, and will, fix your heart if you ask Him and trust Him.

Sometimes, people have physical problems with their heart. In fact, according to three surveys that I checked, heart disease is the number one cause of death in the United States. It seems sensible to treat your heart with respect!

What is the best thing to do for your heart? Learn what you need to do, this can include exercise, diet, weight, many things. Trust God. He tells you be of good courage, and He shall strengthen your heart.

Do find out what science tells you to do, then ask God what of those do you need!

I have noticed that if a pastor talks about people talking during a sermon, the only people who pay attention are the ones who never talk. The people that the pastor wants their attention are too busy thinking about other things to hear what was said.

The same is true for your health. Ask God what changes do you need to make.

> Psalm 31:24 - Be of good courage,
> and He shall strengthen your heart,
> all you who hope in the LORD.

By Patricia L. Whipp

## December 29

What is a supplication? It is a form of prayer. It is usually an earnest plea. It does not have to be in writing, but it can be. Don't be hasty to pray, take time to think about what you are praying, what you want, and what the Word says.

When you want healing, there are times when you will just take authority. But there may be times when you want to pray, and seek God concerning your healing. This is when you need to search the scriptures. I have even asked God for advice concerning prayer and what scriptures to use.

God will give you the advice, and the help needed, to pray appropriately. There are times when you will use several scriptures, and will be formal in your prayer. There are times when, "Lord, HELP," is sufficient, but that is not always true.

When you have sought the Word, formed your supplication, then you have the confidence that God will receive your prayer. With that confidence, you can rest assured that your prayer will be answered.

Praise God for His goodness.

Psalm 6:9 - The LORD has heard my supplication; the LORD will receive my prayer.

## December 30

Man has always searched for the fountain of youth, or the fountain of life. Ponce de Leon left Spain and ended up near America in the 1400s, searching for the fountain of life. This sort of thing has gone on since the fall.

This fountain of youth is also supposed to be a fountain of health. There have been areas with bodies of water around the world where it was felt that healing occurred. We read about at least one of these during the life of Jesus.

According to Proverbs, you have a well of life in you, your mouth. (Proverbs 10:11) What you speak can cause health, and it can cause sickness. Actually, that knowledge occurs many places in the Bible.

Do you talk sickness? "I always get the flu every winter." That is why you have the flu. You give Satan full permission to bring the flu to you. "Every spring my allergies start up." You are saying, "Allergies come to me."

Facts are what you see, what man reports. Truth is what the Bible says. Truth is always stronger than facts. Learn to always speak truth. Learn what the Bible says.

> Proverbs 10:11 - The mouth of the righteous is a well of life, but violence covers the mouth of the wicked.

## December 31

God made promises to Israel. When you have become a Christian, you become heirs of Abraham, and you receive the promises made to Abraham and his seed.

When hard times come, when bad things happen, God will be with you. When you are in a fire, He will protect you. These promises have been made to us. Learn to use them. If you can be convinced that they aren't your promises, then you will not receive the protection promised to you.

Many people are robbed simply because of a lack of knowledge of their rights. God's Words are, "My people are destroyed for a lack of knowledge." You have a choice. You can accept bad things, or you can stand for what is rightfully yours.

Read your Bible, study, and learn.

Receive the promises of God. Learn what is yours. Learn to walk in the fullness of His promises. Trust God, use your authority, and demand your rights.

> Isaiah 43:2 - When you pass through the waters, I will be with you; and through the rivers, they shall not overflow you. When you walk through the fire, you shall not be burned, nor shall the flame scorch you.

# *Appendix*

Salvation Information

Where to Find More Scriptures

Where to Obtain Scripture Cards

Books by Patricia L. Whipp

By Patricia L. Whipp

# *Salvation Information*

Are you born again? Have you made Jesus your Lord and Savior? If you were to die today, do you know that you would go to heaven?

If you are not sure about any of the above questions, then make Jesus your Lord and Savior. How can you do that? Read the confession in the next two paragraphs out loud.

**I confess with my mouth that I believe that Jesus is Lord. I believe in my heart that God has raised Jesus from the dead.**

**I receive Jesus as my Lord and Savior. Thank you God that I now know I am born again.**

The confession which you have just made is taken from the Bible. It is Romans 10:9-10.

Tell someone what you have done. Find a church where people believe in being born again, and where they use and teach the Bible. It is so important to learn what is in the Bible, what God is telling you. It is also good to have fellowship with other people who can help you learn more.

Contact us and let us know that you have now received Jesus as your Lord and Savior. Contact information is available on the following pages.

By Patricia L. Whipp

# *Where to Find More Scriptures*

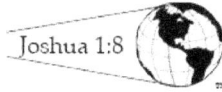

Joshua 1:8

## God's Word Going Forth
PO Box 8015
La Verne, CA 91750

Email: Contact@godswordgoingforth.org

Website: godswordgoingforth.org

If you would like to work on other areas of your life besides healing, you can go to the above website. There are over 140 pages of BibleNotes. From these notes, you can find other scriptures. Examples would be:

Anger
Forgiveness
Body of Christ

These would each have different scriptures listed, as well as other useful information.

Did you receive Jesus as your Lord and Savior on the previous page? Please contact us by email, the website, or a letter to the above address.

We look forward to hearing from you.

By Patricia L. Whipp

# Where to Obtain Scripture Cards

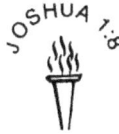

JOSHUA 1:8

**The Printed Word**
PO Box 7734
La Verne CA 91750

Email: CardSets@printedword.org

Website: printedword.org

You can purchase sets of scripture cards on the website listed above. There are 20-60 cards in each set, with a different scripture on each card. Titles include:

Confidence (Power in Your Words)
Fear Not
Wisdom

as well as many more.

Also, at this site you will find books and CDs with scriptures on them. There are scripture card sets in Spanish as well as English.

By Patricia L. Whipp

# *Books by*
# *Patricia L. Whipp*

Following Whom I Serve - KJV

Confessions and Prayers for Daily Living

Healing Is Yours

Healing Devotions

Bits and Pieces Devotions

Following Whom I Serve - NKJ Revised